Stephen B. Strum, M.D.
Robert H. Joseph, M.D.

Diplomates American
Boards of Internal
Medicine and Medical
Oncology

Oncology, Hematology, Internal Medicine
9201 Sunset Boulevard, Suite 201
Los Angeles, California 90069
(213) 550-8076

Members of American
Society of Clinical
Oncology, American
Association of Cancer
Research, American
College of Physicians

A SMALL BUT RAPIDLY GROWING NUMBER OF PHYSICIANS ARE BECOMING AWARE OF A RE-BORN PHILOSOPHY AND PRACTICE OF MEDICINE TERMED "WHOLISTIC". IT EMBRACES RELIGION AND SCIENCE, MIND AND BODY, AND SOUL, AND ENGENDERS A TRANQUILITY OF SPIRIT. RECENTLY IN MY LIFE, I EXPERIENCED SEVERE PAIN AND WITH IT ANXIETY, PANIC AND FEAR. AS I READ ELAN'S BOOK, AN IMMEDIATE IDENTIFICATION WITH THE MAN AND HIS THOUGHTS WAS REALIZED. HIS PHILOSOPHY IS ONE OF HEIGHTENED CONSCIOUSNESS. IT IS A NEW YET AGELESS PHILOSOPHY THAT RELATES NOT ONLY TO HEALING, BUT TO A WAY OF LIVING.

STEPHEN B. STRUM, M.D.

Dear Reader:

You are holding a valuable key to a storehouse of accumulated knowledge and love. Through it, you may realize a better, richer, more fully lived life.

I have written simply, so that the initial meaning is clear. A more sophisticated meaning can flower as you integrate the initial interpretation into your reservoir of experience.

I have permeated my words with energy, so they will work on a deeper and higher level than the mere intellectual and conscious: they are abundant with fertile love so that your own inner love may rise to a full flame enveloping and caressing you with its glow and warmth. They are charged with a healing psychic energy so that your energies will be revitalized. They are enveloped in the light of universal truth so that your enlightenment will shine brighter.

This is more than a "how to" book. This may be a channel and tool of healing...a love of full and joyous life.

In universal love, your
fellow human traveler
and student of life,

Elan Z. Neev

WHOLISTIC HEALING

by Dr. ELAN Z. NEEV

How to harmonize your body, mind and spirit
with life – for freedom, joy, health, beauty,
love, money and psychic powers

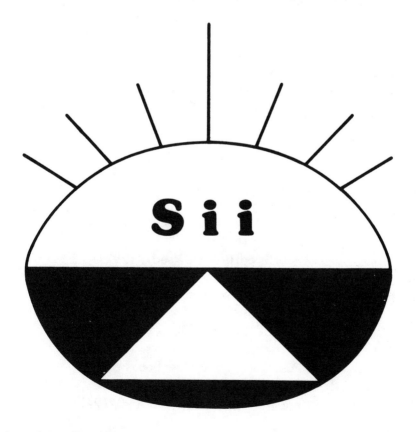

S i i

Ageless Books

L.C. Card No. 77-71152

Self-improvement symbol and
the cover design were
channeled and created
through Elan Z. Neev.

© Elan Z. Neev 1977, 1982, 1993

First edition, 1977 (including a limited ,
exclusive printing of deluxe hard cover,
gold on cloth)
Second edition, 1978
Third edition, 1979
Fourth edition (revised), 1982
Fifth edition (with a very minor revision & an addendum), 1993
Library of Congress Catalog Card Number: 77-71152

ISBN 0-918482- 00-3

Published by Ageless Books
P.O. Box 6300
Beverly Hills, California 90212-1300

DEDICATION

DEDICATED TO ALL MY TEACHERS IN LIFE, THOSE WHO LOVED ME AND THOSE WHO DIDN'T -- ESPECIALLY TO THE LATTER, AS THEY FORCED ME TO RELY UPON MYSELF TO FIND BETTER PATHS.

WHAT ABOUT NUTRITION?
(An added introduction for the health food -minded)

As this book goes into its fourth printing, I feel that some good people need the extra explanation I am about to give. It has to do with food, consciousness, and health.

While the majority of health food store managers and health enthusiasts see very clearly how this book, WHOLISTIC HEALING, belongs with all good health-oriented books, some appear a bit hazy about how a book, which is apparently more about consciousness raising than about health food and supplements, will benefit a health and fitness lover.

Let me, therefore, explain some of my strong views on the subject. When I go into a health food restaurant, I look not only at the menu. I sense the vibrations within the place. If, for example, I note that the owner and the cook are in conflict--or that the waiters are unhappy for any reason--I politely leave. This is because what I term "wellness" is the result of the interaction of all intersecting energies, or vibrations. Wellness is a whole, expressed through harmonious vibrations. Disharmonious vibrations from any source can disturb the harmonious balance.

The best and most healthful food can be damaged on the fundamental vibratory level, and I don't want to ingest health food contaminated by anger. Yet even such contamination can be alleviated by radiating positive vibrations into the food by, for instance, blessing it. Noted nutritionist Dr. Barbara Charis has this to say about that: "Man would exist far better on limited quantities of high quality food, but bless it please. It's very important for people to realize that spiritual nourishment can be obtained through the blessing of food."

If for some reason, however, I am served food which is not perfectly pure, healthful, and in ideal combination, I may bless and enjoy it, if it has been prepared and served with much love and in such a harmonious atmosphere that the good vibrations compensate for the weaknesses of the food. It is all a matter of balance.

The law of balance operates on all levels; food and eating are no exceptions. I would like you to know the master keys to health, wellness, and fulfillment. Even if right now you are more interested in good nutrition than in consciousness, reading this book thoroughly will prepare you for better nutrition and for better results from proper eating! Studying and applying the principles in this book will help you better understand how to use those aspects of harmony and wellness that are behind all good nutrition and healing. You'll then improve your communications with your body and its needs, and more accurately choose the diet which is best for you at different times and under different conditions. (That's right; different people may need different food and supplements at different times.) You'll better understand and know "what and when." With the knowledge imparted in WHOLISTIC HEALING, you can more easily find your way through the maze of NEW AGE diets. You won't get confused as easily, or "taken," and you'll become more skillful in reconciling differences and conflicts. You may even be inspired to combine the best elements from a few diets, add your own ideas flowing to you in inspiration (or Divinely guided), and create your very own, very best healthful eating guides.

Here are a few examples of how you can use the information in this book to support and improve your nutrition. On page 45, I wrote: "Our great task is to learn not to interfere with this natural and spontaneous healing force" (the Great Life Force). I list unnatural foods and drugs as interferences with the flow. Understanding this will immediately give you more motivation to eat naturally, and to replace drugs with healing foods, herbs, vitamins, minerals, and other natural food supplements. The value of eating correctly will be further enhanced when you become aware of the vital life force that can be received through health foods.

Studying Chapter 4, "HEALING DISEASE THE SAFE, NATURAL WAY", will assist you in getting the maximum value from your dietary regimen. Page 53, e.g., mentions how you can use food and drink "to focus powerful healing energies on ailments or conditions."

WHOLISTIC HEALING/WHAT ABOUT NUTRITION

As I discussed in the chapter about Cosmic Aikido, everything is energy, which of course includes food. By better understanding the nature of energy, you'll be better guided toward pure and high energy food that will raise your energy on all levels. You'll better understand how fresh and natural food that has been grown, sold, prepared, and eaten in an environment of good vibrations, can make you become not only healthier and more powerful, but more spiritual as well. And you'll also understand better how developing your spiritual nature and awareness can help you eat better. Spiritual food and natural food are a perfect combination!

In a forthcoming book called COLOR LIVING^R, I've explained in detail the theory that eating by the rainbow (that is, eating foods and drinking juices that represent all the colors of the rainbow) is a sure way to ascertain a good nutritional balance with high and complete vibratory rapport with Mother Nature and Father God. I invite contributions from researchers and/or writers who are experienced in the application of colors to specific areas such as nutrition, psychology, healing, and environments. Those contributions could be included as an anthology in COLOR LIVING^R.

According to one of the secrets of the Holy Hebrew Kabala, as taught by the 18th century Rabbi Moshe Hayeem Lutzato in his book DA'AT TEVOONOT (Knowledge of Wisdom), published in B'nai Brak, Israel--Man was created potentially perfect. However, Man was created as a vessel into which he could put whatever he chose with the power of free will given to him. Man has the choice to damage his potentially perfect

vessel, as Adam and Eve did, and eat the wrong food, literally and figuratively, and thus suffer the consequences.
But Man also has the capacity to learn and repent, eat
the right things and perfect himself; elevating himself
thus to better life and eventually to God-like eternal life!

Then, truly perfected, as desired by the Creator
from the beginning, Man would eat from the Tree of Life,
transcending death, illness, atrophy, entrophy, and
destructive thoughts and actions. Men and women then
will enjoy the light in paradise for ever and ever...

In this exciting transitory period, when people of
various religions predict the imminent appearance of the
Messiah, you can make modest but important preparation,
regardless of your beliefs: Purify and strengthen your own
vessel, your own body, your own personality. At least
you will thus bring about your own inner redemption.

At this stage of your life--if your primary path to
the good life is already health and nutrition--I suggest
you also read and apply WHOLISTIC HEALING. It will
help you benefit more fully from your food and from
everything that Nature gives you and you give Nature.

The Author

AN ENDORSEMENT BY A NUTRITIONAL AUTHORITY
"As a nutritional researcher for 20 years and as
a graduate of one of Dr. Neev's classes, I wholeheart-
edly recommend WHOLISTIC HEALING for all people
who are sincerely interested in good health and wholesome living. It will prepare you for more effective
giving and receiving of blessings."

Dr. Barbara Charis, Charis Holistic Center, WLA, Ca.

TYPICAL COMMENTS FROM READERS

Introductory note

The Kabala (often spelled Kabbalah) channels an infinitely deep and wide understanding of the secrets of life on all levels and in all dimensions, as inspired by the mystical exploration of the Scriptures. It literally means in Hebrew "receiving." Such knowledge, such intelligence, can only be received by those who are receptive. Receptiveness can be developed by trust and faith. Receptiveness can be inspired by the enthusiasm of others.

I want you to believe in this book, because I want you to receive all that I am worthy of sharing with you, some of which may be Kabala knowledge. The more you believe that the principles described in WHOLISTIC HEALING can work for you, the more they indeed will! The more you trust in the Divine power within you and in the Universe, the more you can do for yourself and others.

Following are some quotes from letters of readers who developed enthusiasm through experiencing this book. You can feast on this energy, becoming more open to receiving all the blessings that may come to you through owning and reading WHOLISTIC HEALING. Then, through your enriched love energy, you will radiate multiplied blessings back to those readers and to the entire creation. We will all, then, evolve toward greater experience of the ONENESS and the infinite GOOD.

Different individuals may have different needs and preferences at different times. A stubborn skeptic, or an individual whose faith was depleted by failure and suffering, may need the build-up offered by the following barrage of fan letters. The repetitious phrases of enthusiasm and love can be very therapeutic for them, like affirmations. For a person "sold" on wholistic healing, so much praise can feel like an overdose of medicine. If you are such an individual, please bear with me, and, by all means, skip the comments and plunge into the body and soul of the book!

"...I am presently attending Pennsylvania State University with a major in Nutrition. These past few months I have been becoming increasingly interested in the concept of Wholism, but more specifically--wholistic healing.

I was in a bookstore one day looking for books pertaining to wholistic health when I came across your book. I was unaware at the time of the great impact this book was to make on me.

Although I had not done much previous reading on this subject before I read WHOLISTIC HEALING , many of the ideas which you wrote about confirmed the thoughts which have been developing in my own mind over the last several weeks. Naturally, my craving to find out more about wholistic healing has increased tremendously.

It is for this reason why I felt compelled to write this letter. I not only wanted to express my thanks to you for writing this tremendous book, but also to ask if any information could be sent to me about the Wholistic Self-Improvement Training which was mentioned in your book. I feel an urgency to explore any avenue that will help me find my 'whole self.'"

Lisa Werst

"...I recommend that you get a copy of WHOLISTIC HEALING by Dr. Elan Z. Neev and read it carefully. The book goes beyond what a casual perusal of the title might indicate. Both book and author have a 'good feel'...If the book stirs up something in you, I suggest that you telephone him, and possibly go and meet him."

Col. Robert B. Emerson, pastor, THE GROUP - a non-profit religious group researching biophysics and parapsychology

"...it's just what I needed at the time - reaffirming many inner truths. I don't know if it was parapsychological or what - but I felt a healing light in my stomach - just where I store all my pain."

Robin Siegel

WHOLISTIC HEALING/TYPICAL COMMENTS

"Once again Dr. Neev demonstrated to me his divine gift of safely channeling the high wisdom and energies of the Hierarchy to all, this time through the printed word. This book imparts healing and knowledge not only semantically but also subtly, through pulsation of power and tenderness experienced within the reader as light, color, sound, temperature, and whole pictures."

Dr. Judith Drake

"...I've been touched by your words. I am now more free; I am more me. I can now share. My unfinished book will . . . be written. Thank you."

Rochelle Rabin

"WHOLISTIC HEALING transformed my life. I've avidly studied many self-help books, but this is the first time I've been guided to a book that has such a powerful effect as a synthesis of inspiration, practical step-by-step advice, exciting entertainment, and real love energy. . . I've used it to heal severe headaches and emotional and financial pain as well as a textbook to help me teach and counsel. I have even slept with the book under my pillow for the sphere and the pyramid energies!"

Ruth M. Guernsey

"I have been a metaphysical student for many years and although I am most familiar with all of your teaching, I find in your book an inspiration to apply the teaching to my own life and circumstances more than I have ever before."

Sara M. Gerst

WHOLISTIC HEALING/TYPICAL COMMENTS

"Dr. Neev provides excellent guidance for the direct under-standing of the depth and potential of one's own mind. It represents a fresh and promising way to introduce students to vital metaphysical issues for self-improvement and problem solving. Rarely has such a clear and brilliant picture been presented. We can learn to be both creative and spontaneous which is a remarkable flow of the mind/body process. Through these understandings we can enjoy more success and confidence in all aspects of our lives, in our work, in our relation-ships and in our own personal growth."

Bruce D. Wasserman, Biochemist and Silva Mind Control Instructor

"Blessings on you for writing such a book. At age 78 and alone, I not only want it to refer to, but need it and am glad my friend found it."

Charlene Ramalho

"We humbly present that it has been by the Lord's grace that we have come across your address.... will be an invaluable asset to our inquiring minds."

Kubanda P.M., Sserulanda Nsulo Yobulamu Institution, Uganda, Africa

"...your book ...was at a bookstore in Calgary. I might say an out of the way book store. It's great! I love it! I've been pass-ing it around to friends, but not for long as I refer to it a lot.... I can't seem to get enough of it. A day doesn't pass that I don't read some part of it."

Klaus and Lynda Tenter, Alberta, Canada

"Your book WHOLISTIC HEALING is just wonderful. As an Israeli Yoga teacher I integrated your teachings into my work. It certainly enhances what I share with my students. You should translate it into Hebrew. People here are ready and thirsty for a book such as yours. Any chance you'll be lecturing and teaching here, too?"

S.M., Israel

"Salutation and adoration! Sir, I have been influenced very much about your grand teaching...want to come down to learn. I have full hopes to share your unique teachings... "

Dr. K.D. Chauhan, Jagdishnagar Society, India

"Elan, I felt very close to you and admired and loved you and thought you did a great deal of good to further the cause of cosmic or universal unity, or good for all mankind. I very thoughtfully read and finished studying your very deep and wonderful book...I did enjoy it and learned so much I feel like a new man, and will re-read it and put it to use and practice it ...all the wonderful instructions. It is one of the most uplifting and inspiring books to read !
Elan, I am 84 years old and I have seen lots of life and worldly doings. I do want to take your Wholistic Self-Improvement Training, however... "

David Griffith

"I have become aware of the fact that if I am going to turn my life around to be successful, I will have to do something for myself. I am presently in prison. "

Chris Brown, Sierra Conservation Center, Department of
Correction

"Your pictures tell more than words can say! "

Edith Halbert

WHOLISTIC HEALING/TYPICAL COMMENTS

"Thank you so much for the copy of your book, <u>WHOLISTIC</u> <u>HEALING</u>. I have enjoyed reading it very much and <u>know that it</u> <u>will</u> bring comfort and inspiration to many. I have told friends about your work and have given them the information to get in touch with you, which I hope they do."

Gayla Claes

"I have just finished your book, <u>WHOLISTIC HEALING</u>. <u>...as you can see by my ordering two of your tapes ... have</u> <u>gotten a great deal out of it!</u>"

(Mrs.) Jean M. Starks

"I just don't know how to express what I felt while reading it. In fact, I will probably read it again and again, it was that inspiring to me. I teach Expanded Awareness classes here in Syracuse, N.Y. area professionally, and healing is one of the subjects I teach. Your ideas are not new to me, but the manner in which you express them and the refinements were, and very enlightening...I would love to take part in your Wholistic Self-Improvement Course. Do you ever take your course to the East?

Carol Ann Porter

"I finished reading your book and I find it fantastic. Have been a metaphysical student for about 25 years and have not yet found a self-help book as yours. I am a senior citizen working as a volunteer for Damien Simpson who is on Channel 52 "Psychic Phenomena, The World Beyond"... Maybe you can get on his program as a guest. . . . Would like to be put on your mailing list and will bring some friends to one of your classes or lectures. Thank you again for your very helpful book. I stayed awake all night finishing it. . . ."

Roberta Winant

WHOLISTIC HEALING/TYPICAL COMMENTS

"My wife and I have just finished listening to you on New Dimension Radio. We are excited and would like very much to study and learn with you."

Larry Anderson

"I heard you on KALW - San Francisco. What an inspiration! Thank you. Would you please send me a copy of your book WHOLISTIC HEALING? Enclosed is a check for $12 which I hope will cover the cost."

John Corgiat

"HARMONY GROVE loves you. Your recent presentation here was received enthusiastically by those attending your lecture. Some of the comments were 'witty,' 'interesting,' 'easy to understand,' 'well-spoken,' 'helpful,' and 'motivating.' One of our members who is notorious for sleeping through everything actually was awake the whole time and came away excited by what you had to say. My own comment is that you brought love, joy, and Truth to HARMONY GROVE.

Many of our members - including this one - have responded most favorably to your book, WHOLISTIC HEALING. I marvel that so much Truth was imparted so painlessly. I found the book highly readable, practical, and applicable to many aspects of the quest for physical, emotional, and spiritual harmony. I recommend the book and you most highly. In fact, I am urging the manager of our bookstore to order copies for sale. I feel that our members and visitors should have the opportunity to find your path to self-awareness and development. Thank you for sharing so much of yourself with us. So often those who 'have it, hoard it.' You are most generous to share it, and I can personally attest that you very definitely 'have it.'

Helene M. Guthrie

WHOLISTIC HEALING/TYPICAL COMMENTS

"I saw very briefly a copy of ...WHOLISTIC HEALING. This would appear to be a very unique book with very helpful, practical knowledge."

J. Henly

"I feel in harmony with everything you talk about in your book. I am a Rebirther studying wholistic health and communications.... I feel you would be a success here. I suggest you come over and offer your training."

Catherine Piscitello,
Hawaii

"One of my goals is to be able to attend your class. I have had a burning desire for years to serve mankind in a positive, constructive way -- that each takes the responsibility for himself. Your book...has opened many new avenues for me. Thanks for caring and sharing. Please send the following Self Improvement tapes:#5,7,8."

S/Lovita Presley

"I thought I'd drop you a short note while ordering your book for a friend. A friend of mine had sent me a copy just yesterday and I can already feel the effects on my life. I am healing from an illness, and being able to use some of your techniques has helped me tremendously. Please send me an additional hard back copy of WHOLISTIC HEALING. A friend of mine owns a book store. He was reading my copy of your book and had several people interested in obtaining it."

Mary Clark

WHOLISTIC HEALING/TYPICAL COMMENTS

"We are seriously interested in your Publication which we strongly objectify to consider for possible adoption and use in our dual Education Programme, as well as for use and sale at our University Public Service Library and Bookshop respectively."

Dr. Ricardo Solomon, Principal, Mid Western University,
Republic of Guyana

"The book has been lent to me by a friend, and I think it was bought at the Chalk Farm Nutrition Center, London. I think the book is an excellent and realistic synthesis of many spiritual ideas, and its ideas apply to the ordinary lives of ordinary people. When I first picked the book up, I found it very uplifting, as it seemed to talk about many things I had come to believe were true, but had not read about anywhere else. So often spiritual books seem to have nothing to do with reality, but your book shows a wise understanding of reality. I particularly liked the pictures."

John Nyyte, England

"...I found your book in a health store in Hollywood. As soon as I saw the book it attracted me powerfully, so that I had to buy it. Let me tell you now that I have read it, it is really good. Every page is enlightening and written with a good sense of humor. Whenever I suffer from tensions or fears, I get myself inside the energizer and pyramid. I feel wonderful now. It is a great book! The world needs a lot of people like you. Keep up the work, dear Doctor, and help as much as possible all the unfortunate and unprivileged people who have nothing, not even health. Write more, flow the markets and bookstores with all your books. I know there are many souls who want to be helped."

Fanny Stillman

"Your book is exceptional! Through it I have made a beautiful new step in my awareness, and I want to say thank-you.... Enclosed money is for your book, and an extra amount if you will please send another one for a friend of mine."

Farrell

"I have just read your book WHOLISTIC HEALING for the third time. TERRIFIC! I also bought 3 copies (all they had) for others.
I have been a metaphysical student for about 4 years. Everything I have learned so far is in your book in less than 100 pages. Bless you. I especially like your graphic style of writing and illustrations. I now have a book that I can recommend as being interesting, easy to read and short. They won't read it if you tell them it would help them. The only suggestion I might make is the fact that wholistic healing or higher consciousness does take time and effort. You make it sound so easy.

Jane Krafka

"...the maxim 'good things come in small packages' applies here."

Newspaper review by
Rustie Brown

"I would like to order 10 copies of WHOLISTIC HEALING ... you can be sure my one and only copy of the book has been shared a lot! These first 10 copies probably won't be enough--so you'll be hearing from me."

Ms. Monnie L. Kindy, M.T.
Massagologist

"...A friend who lives there presented the book WHOLISTIC HEALING by Elan Neev. In reading this book I developed a strong desire to follow some of its precepts, and to present this book to some of my friends. I need about 5 copies."

Lewis A. Albee

"...what a wonderful book. It's one of the best I've ever read in the field. It's loaded! There's so much good in it. I must and will read it again and again. I also think your tape #12 is beautiful, the music I enjoy and your meditation also is soothing and very pleasant. I love your voice. Rendering it you have something beautiful in you. I can't explain it, but I know it's good.

My grandson, Michael, and I have been listening to your tape , and I gave him your book."

Michael Fecko

"There isn't a day that goes by that I don't use at least one of the techniques from WHOLISTIC HEALING for self-improvement. I feel at this point that I even have more to gain from some of your tapes."

Mary Clark

"I purchased your book on Wholistic Healing in Phoenix two years ago. I enjoyed it - and especially the colors of orange and blue. They are the two colors that I feel very strongly about.... There definitely does need to be better communication in the international organizations and in the world."

Katrina T. Blank

"I have just completed reading Dr. Neev's book, WHOLISTIC HEALING. I was very impressed with it. I have a keen interest in caring for the physical body in a 'whole' way, and Dr. Neev's techniques felt right for me. I initially bought the book because I looked at the picture on the back cover and thought, 'Wow, I know this man.' There was an awareness that he had something to share with me. Anyway, what I am writing for is some information on Wholistic Self-Improvement Training courses...."

Darleen Ward

WHOLISTIC HEALING/TYPICAL COMMENTS

"Your book WHOLISTIC HEALING has opened up a whole world for me. I had recently been on a path of self destruction, doing things I knew I would regret and wondering why I was allowing those things to happen. Now I realize what I was doing was a diversion away from the Christ-self, a separation of energy. The love-light has brought my center back into focus.

I am eighteen years young and have grown up in a very oppressive environment. I am learning and growing spiritually, but I feel a yearning to have some personal help and guidance. I feel love speaking through you to the children of the New Age. Thank you for writing a beautiful book that brings love to our brothers."

Rebecca Carpenter

"I have read your book WHOLISTIC HEALING and am re-reading and studying it and applying its principles in my life. There are too many books that promise us 'how to' achieve something but are filled with countless words, double-talk, dissertations and theories - empty promises. Your book truly does tell us 'how to' achieve, with working methods that must succeed when used with a correct attitude and motivation. Your spontaneity, enthusiasm and sincerity to share the truths you know with others for expansion of their awareness, comes across loud and clear through your communication in the book.

My inner self attuned... and I cried with you - a waterfall of tears for a dear family of four. Then I cried extra for two beautiful people and that which you did not mention in your book. I like your style for its clarity and your sense of humor is delicious - don't know what else to call it."

Anna Tomin

"I borrowed it (the book) and immediately got 'into' it. I took it to Venice Beach and shortly thereafter found myself in awe by what you had written. I felt spellbound and could not put down your book until it was finished!!! Upon completion, I felt One with the Ocean; Universe; a feeling of joy; Rebirth - a new

WHOLISTIC HEALING/TYPICAL COMMENTS

concept of Life without further physical limitations; my self-
confidence pulsates within the veins of my senses!!"

Christina

"What a beautiful book....WHOLISTIC HEALING. Reading
the book, a feeling of Love overcame me so much that if you had
been close I would have given you a hug - but instead I hugged the
book...a book to treasure. Please send me COSMIC DOODLINGS
and Tape 3."

Clara Okon

"WHOLISTIC HEALING is a New Age psychological and psychic
primer...highly imaginative and original... very intense, very direct,
very to the point."

Review by Stanley Krippner, Ph.D. (former president of Association
of Humanistic Psychology), Chief Editor of Advances in Parapsychological Research

"Several months ago I found your book at a friend's house...I
received it 3rd hand. I found it enjoyable reading, unpretentious and
amusing. It answered some of my questions in a way I found appealing to
my imagination. I accepted some of it, rejected most of it, and put it
away for several months...
    In a dream I found myself lying in a large bed, desolate and alone.
The pain was intense and I curled up in a ball on the edge of the bed...
I didn't know how to stop the pain ...Suddenly someone put their arms
around me in a very tender movement. I thought it was my mother and
turned to thank her. I was shocked. It was a healer. I was momentarily
frightened but a word was spoken, the embrace tightened, and I felt a wave
of unconditional love like I have never experienced: not to possess or mani-
pulate, but to soothe and heal. I trusted him and the pain went away!
    ... I was profoundly moved by my dream and felt very grateful to
the healer. I didn't know who he was...and I found myself haunted by the
image of that man, the man I dreamed, incorporeal and unreal. I loved

him. . . It probably comes as no surprise to you...but I was shocked when, today, on impulse, I pulled your book off the shelf to discover on the back cover the healer in my dream!

I guess I was more moved by your book than I cared to admit to myself. I guess I am writing to thank you for a dream...for the experience of unconditional love...for the experience of trust..."

Tia Claassen

"...wonderful book. It gave me a good outlook on life in general, and I feel rejuvenated!"

Evelyn Siegel

"I got your book at a health food store that a homeopathic doctor recommended to me...I was at the Farmers Market Co-op to buy some health supplies and saw this book and thought it would give me some peace of mind... I never finished reading your book the first time due to my lack of concentration and feeling of dis-ease, as my teacher now tells me. But it did help me then to get over my feeling of fear and hate. ...I have now finished this book and have learned not only how to just relax, but also how to deal with my loved ones, my work, and myself, and how to be a better person... Your book was of more help to me this time than when I first purchased it, because the situation now is more life threatening. Yes, a crisis in one's life definitely causes or inspires a change! I hope that I will be able to raise my consciousness above and beyond so that these painful experiences will not have to happen again. I know I will grow and learn from all that happens as long as I have the courage to admit things about myself...I WISH I HAD FINISNED THE BOOK SOONER...Keep it coming!"

Joanne Smits

WHOLISTIC HEALING/TYPICAL COMMENTS

" I was very excited to read your book WHOLISTIC HEALING, which I received from my neighbor Shoshana..... You conducted a work-shop at her place when you were in Israel. I and Shoshana study the book together sometimes, and are very impressed.....Today I understand that I brought upon myself my illness..... It's the result of my way of living....I beleive you can help.... " (translated from Hebrew)

Danniel, Tel-Aviv, Israel

" It's 'pumkin hour' and I have just finished reading your book WHOLISTIC HEALING. I bought it today from an isolated little shop called 'Styles and Styles' in an isolated little city called 'Hamilton', in an isolated little country called 'New Zealand'.

In many ways your book didn't tell me anything that I didn't already know (about holism and The Self, that is). And yet, I have the feeling, that while this may be true, I have also learned something – but it's something that can't be put into words.

In short, I enjoyed, appreciated, was interested, feel enthusiastic about your book. But there is something else: I really savoured the humour - expressed in words and drawings - and the lesson that went with it. I see humour as an absolute essential for healthy living. And I see being able to laugh at oneself as a crucial facet of that 'essentia-lity'. And yet, there are so many people who can't laugh at themselves!

I see your book as offering both the opportunity and introduction for 'Self to meet the self'; for people to meet and form an intimate relationship with someone they perhaps have never REALLY met or known before - namely themselves. The benefits of such a meeting are obvious. May I take the opportunity to order five copies of WHOLISTIC HEALING...."

Megan-Jane Johnstone
New Zealand

"Your book WHOLIOSTIC HEALING has opened all of me to the awareness of new age thinking. Thank you for sharing your strength and knowledge.... I found your book in a library 'by chance' as I was passing by the shelf of new books. I would like to purchase a copy to re-read and share with friends.

Until we meet in human flesh in this life or another, let us share the divine love light through our ENERGY TRANSCEIVERS. I am a long time beleiver in non-traditional, non-verbal communication."

Rosemary Gabriele

CONTENTS

CHAPTER 1

DEFINING THE INDEFINABLE

Words, words, words, words...

We in the Western world are accustomed to labeling and defining everything. It makes us feel secure. It gives us the illusion of a guarantee that something is exactly as someone who labeled it meant it to be. And we expect it to be that way. We take it for granted to be as defined.

Is there anything wrong with it? Not if we take words and definitions as merely tools of communication, as a means to simplify life. But the moment we let those words become more than a tool -- at the moment we let words and definitions become our masters -- we are in for trouble. Why? Because words are limited. They are not the WHOLE truth. They are limited by our intellectual mind and by our five senses. They are limited by our experience and level of understanding and perceiving. They are limited by our fears and prejudices. WORDS ARE NOT THINGS. WORDS ARE NOT FEELINGS. WORDS ARE NOT THOUGHTS. WORDS ARE NOT ACTION. They are at best an attempt to describe something subjectively perceived or conceived in a way objectively understood. The more similar the subjective experience of the person hearing or reading the words is to that of the speaker or writer of these words, the more complete the communication.

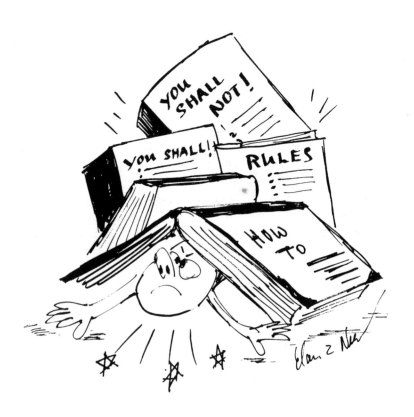

The problems with words arise when the following things happen:

A.   When we experience the words sent quite differently from what their sender intended, because words can mean different things to different people.

B.   When we perceive reality (and fantasy, which IS a part of reality) only through the words and definitions we are accustomed to, instead of perceiving it as directly as possible... being ready to modify or abandon our old definitions according to the experience of the here and now as a flowing, ever-changing part of the unity of past and future.

C.   When we attempt to force our definition on others.

D.   When we blindly, or because of fear or laziness, accept the definition of others as the only possible truth.

In other words, when definitions, dogmas and words become more important than the spontaneous experience, we may become slaves to the tyranny of words and stifle the flow of life through us or those under our influence.

If, right now, you feel frustrated because you do not understand everything I am saying right away, you are simply proving to yourself, through experience, some of the problems with words. This is why in my classes and private consultations there is more emphasis on the inner experience than on words and definitions. However, because you and I are presently communicating through the printed medium, we have to be content with words as the main tools of communication. But, even though you may not hear my voice right now nor feel my touch (unless you are an advanced psychic), my words may channel some energy to you, for your enlightenment and healing. You may absorb this benevolent energy without being aware of it. The awareness of what you absorbed may come later. As you digest the intelligence conveyed through me to you, expel what your Higher Self judges to be excessive for you or unsuitable for your particular being. Store for further use data that you may not be ready for right now. Integrate into your life all which you are ready for as it flowers within you, nourished by your own roots and resources.

Communication problems: defining the spiritual with the intellectual

As we have seen, it is difficult to convey our experiences to others via words. It is even more difficult to convey someone else's experience to others.   The communication tends to lose its closeness to the original experience -- and consequently its accuracy -- as it is passed from one person to another.   It is like, but worse than, a photo of a photo of a photo of a person, or a copy of a copy of a copy of a tape recording of a live voice.

Our communication difficulties multiply a great deal when we try to communicate to someone with words a spiritual experience we encounter.   How can we expect to adequately use the language of the five senses and the intellect to describe something which is beyond their reach?   It is a common problem I experience with novices and new students and clients who haven't yet developed a strong spiritual base or who haven't yet been aware of their spiritual experiences: they often become impatient or frustrated when they attempt to grasp the spiritual world with their intellectual minds and physical tools.

Yet, to effect any meaningful change, such as healing of the body, mind or conditions around us -- intellectual understanding is not enough.   We do not learn to drive a car merely by learning all about driving a car.   We must drive it.   We must experience it directly.   And even then, at first we are very conscious and deliberate with every decision and movement.   And we spend a great deal of energy translating intellectual data and our perceptions into movement of the steering wheel, the pedals, and the blinkers.   Often we are unduly tense and anxious, but once we accumulate sufficient experience, once we are familiar with the road and the vehicle through direct and whole experience rather than through merely intellectual knowledge or the observation of another person's driving, it becomes easier and easier.   Only as we take full responsibility for driving the vehicle (without depending upon the instructor to bail us out in an emergency), can we have peace of mind while driving, to the point of being spontaneous.   Then we can enjoy carefree driving with a minimum expenditure of energy.   We drive almost automatically as our mind is free to think, plan, imagine.   Yet, our awareness becomes whole and vast, like radar scanning effortlessly.   And, if an emergency occurs, our radar flashes the warning to us as we focus the energy we saved and stored, enabling us to take swift and correct action.

Of course, this is the ideal situation.   The freer and more aware the person, the better the radar and the more effective the action.   In fact, part of the Oneness self-improvement training I offer includes psychic driving.   But you will find, I am sure, that even without taking this training, you drive better if you are relaxed.   And you'll find that the energies you save while relaxing are abundantly available when you need to make a swift move.   And the clearer your own energy channels are (your mind and body), the better you can channel creative energies for any purpose with minimum fatigue and wear and tear on your system. This is another secret of Wholistic health.

Like driving, only by total direct and personal experience -- only by taking full responsibility for your action and reaction from within you and without -- can you experience the spiritual. The rewards are great, both psychically and materially.

Transcending the physical limitations of the five senses

The key to Wholistic healing is learning to rise above the material world. That does not mean renouncing the material nature. On the contrary: we must fully accept all there is in order to be able to release all and expand our awareness beyond our intellectual and academic horizons. There is more to life than we are able to perceive with our five senses and to understand through the conscious, intellectual mind. There is more to nature than science is able to explain. Science is confined to what it can prove under controlled laboratory conditions, to what it has discovered. But the vast world that has not yet been discovered and proven by science is not non-existent just because a dissertation or a textbook has not yet been written on it. It exists whether we see it or not; whether we under-stand it or not; whether we prove it or not; whether the majority believes in it or not; whether the "authorities" have approved of it or not.

The whole objective reality is independent of our ability to perceive it. The sooner we humbly accept the limitations of our conscious perception and human intellectual understanding, the sooner we can focus the life energies diverted and saved from the intellectual and emotional wandering onto our unlimited intuitive knowingness. In other words, if we admit we don't know and understand everything there is, and that there is a lot more to life than meets the eye, we are ready to let go of the insistence on knowing, defining and understanding intellectually and through our five senses. Because this insistence can be futile. This insistence can be constricting. This insistence can cause disease of the body and mind, and disaster in business and human relations. This insistence can block healing.

The next step, after we stop insisting on a logical, intellectual explanation -- or any explanation at all -- is to allow our fancy to flow free. As Albert Einstein said, "Imagination is more important than knowledge." To facilitate this flow of our imagination, we are to free our body and mind from any preconceived ideas or restrictions. The more we are able to relax both mind and body and forget them, the more we are able to release our imagination and receive inspiration from our creative subconscious and from Higher Intelligence. This inspiration may be what we need for self-healing, healing of others, healing of problems of life in general. It may come to us as a realization of what and how to do something constructive, or it may guide us on the unconscious level toward spontaneous healing or fulfillment of our needs and goals on all levels.

Meditation is one powerful and safe way of achieving this freedom from our body and intellectual mind as we allow communication with our innermost -- our highest -- to flow. This flow can be translated into perfect health, into immunity and protection, into good relations and happiness, into wisdom and creativity, into psychic and healing powers, into love and fulfillment, into success and prosperity.

Transcending meditation and some affirmations

Sit comfortably with your spine straight, your feet flat on the ground, and your palms up in your lap...or lie straight on your back. Stare fixedly into the sunburst-like oval symbol on the cover of this book. Know that this symbol, comprising some of the most potent energy channeling shapes and symbols, is a Love Energy Transceiver. Know that the seven rays irradiate you with divine healing love-light in the intensity and color combination most beneficial for your individual being...mind, soul and body. Observe the serene oval shape: an egg-like symbol of rebirth, rejuvenation, peace, and harmony. Note the ocean of life within it, and the white pyramid of perfect balance, divine order, healing, and focusing of creative energies. Feel the warm orange love-light caress the exposed parts of your skin, and then your entire body as it permeates it. Etch the image of the Love Energy Transceiver of Self-Improvement in your mind and imagine it with your eyes closed. Know it is out there in space, even if you don't see it. Imagine it pulsating like a big, loving heart. Every time it expands, it engulfs you with relaxing, healing, loving orange light which gently removes all tension and disharmony. Feel your own heart pulsating in harmony with the great Love Energy Transceiver, spreading love, harmony, and peaceful relaxation through your arteries to every cell in your body. Know that you are getting in tune with the celestial rhythm of the universe.

Give yourself to this whole life rhythm. Let go and experience the glowing warmth of the great life force lovingly flowing throughout your being -- freeing it, freeing it, freeing it.... As your physical body becomes l o o s e and totally relaxed, as your restless intellectual and emotional mind ceases to worry and argue, you become still. If some thoughts keep harassing you, occupy your brain with the mantra asserting your responsibility to yourself and your development from within: "self-improvement, self-improvement, self-improvement".... Then feel the spontaneous urge to merge with the ocean of life as the potent Love Energy Transceiver of Self-Improvement magnetizes you toward it. Feel your awareness willingly and longingly rising toward that all-encompassing love transceiver. Feel your awareness getting closer and closer to it until all you can see is the bright white light of the pyramid (or tent of peace) as you enter it.

Now image yourself standing amidst this divine pyramid of white love-light, and imagine you can see and feel an even more intense laser beam of white light rising from the floor of the pyramid up into your groin and through your spine, revitalizing your central nervous system and psychic centers, up through your throat and the top of your head into the center of the ceiling of your pyramid. As you raise your eyes to follow it, see the light beam rising through the ceiling of the pyramid. Now take in a very deep and slow breath of white love energy through your nostrils. Know it hooks onto the Infinite Intelligence. Hold your breath as long as you comfortably can, allowing a spontaneous draught of healing, relaxing, enlightening energy from above. Then, as you s l o w l y release your breath, follow with your eyes and sensations the divine, creative intelligence flowing down through the beam of light, through your brain (100% enlightened and revitalized), and down your spine...pushing down all toxins of mind, soul, and body...all tension and anxiety...all pain and its causes... down through the shaft and into your feet, and into the floor.... As you release and empty your being from all constrictions, the light from above fills the space with the heavenly calm of white love-light. Focus effortlessly all your senses on the white shaft of light in the center of your being, affirming basically the following: "I am centered, I am free, I am grounded. My feet are on the ground safely and firmly planted, but my soul and awareness can rise infinitely. I accept me. I love me. I accept life and its lessons. I do not and will not try to escape life's lessons, not even the painful ones. I can safely let go of my physical shell, knowing I will return in due time, or, whenever it is important for my well-being, with further energies and instructions for my body and personality to make them whole. I trust my Higher Self. I know it will safely guide me out and back. It knows all because it is one with all. I need not worry, need not interfere. I am still, I am still. I am still. I am still...."

Then, just sit there or recline with your spine straight, and enjoy. You may blank out, or you may have a dream-like experience. But even if you are not conscious or understanding of what you have experienced, know you have experienced something beyond your five senses. Know you are better for that.

If, at first you find it difficult to remember and follow (and by no means do you need to follow it to the letter -- you may be guided to a method more suitable for your individuality), you may tape-record and play it. As you practice meditation, it will work for you better and better. Very soon you and others will notice the beauty and calmness glowing through and from you, and the enlarged sensitivity, awareness, wisdom, creativity, and energy.

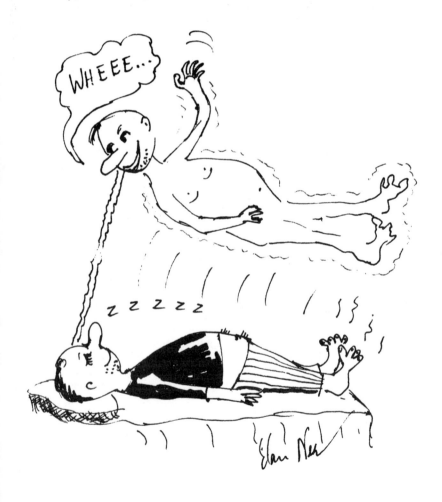

CHAPTER 2

HOW TO TURN PROBLEMS INTO OPPORTUNITIES

<u>The best school: the compulsory school of life</u>

One of the best ways to Wholistic health is total acceptance of life as a series of lessons. This attitude will automatically remove much of the strain and stress of everyday life and of the painful experiences of the past or the dread of tomorrow.

Some of us may not choose to learn. Some of us wish and try to quit the school of life. But, you see, there is no way out. If we try to escape a lesson, we must meet it again, and again, and again...until we face it and learn. It is like the old joke about a mediocre American singer who thought he was the greatest. He sang an aria to an Italian audience. They called for an encore. He sang the aria again. They demanded another encore. He sang again and again and again. His pride in the apparent enthusiasm of his audience at last turned into fatigue and suspicion, when they insisted on more singing. So he asked his audience, "I know I am the greatest, but still, don't you get tired hearing me sing the same song over and over again?" "Yes, we are very tired of hearing you, and it's painful to the ears," said a spokesman for the sophisticated musical audience, "but we want you to sing it over and over again until you sing it right!"

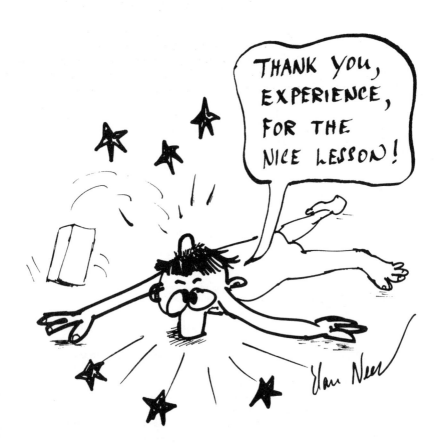

So it is with our painful lessons of life. We must repeat them over and over and over again until we play them right. If we try to escape from a painful relationship in love or business, we will be experiencing new relationships with the same problems and the same pain over and over again. There is no escape: even if we run away and evade new relationships for the fear of repeated pain, we cannot escape the pain. Because we take it with us. And the longer we fight it, the deeper the pain entrenches itself in our systems. If we try to suppress it, it builds up compression and intensity that eats us from within. We may temporarily appear to succeed in suppressing the pain (and the anger or guilt that often accompanies it with an evil sneer), but the most we may do is push it into our subconscious where it sabotages our very foundations, underground and in the dark, from whence it may leap on us any second with destructive violence. The physical result may be anything from indigestion to ulcers, headaches, cancer, heart failure, or strokes, to name a few. Mental results may vary from mental fatigue, temper tantrums, nervous collapses, mania, and such ilk.

If we try to kill the pain with drugs and alcohol, or hypnosis, or even meditation or prayer...it will rise again stronger, and we'll need greater and greater doses of pain killers which also may be destroying our organism or mental and spiritual balance and harmony with nature. We may even become "religious" or "spiritual" freaks, frantically and fanatically wasting life trying to deny reality and its pleasures from ourselves and others around us. Even if we succeed in killing our physical bodies through suicide or self-inflicted disease, according to spiritual teachings, we will still have to return (reincarnate) to suffer the same pain over and over again until we face it, listen to it, accept it and learn from it. ONLY BY LEARNING FROM A PAINFUL PROBLEM CAN WE RELEASE OURSELVES FROM IT.

Unveiling the blessing in disguise

I believe everything that happens to us is for a reason, because life is an unbroken chain of cause and effect. Thus, even a painful experience is for a reason. And since every experience is an opportunity for learning and growth, every problem, mistake, failure, pain, and obstacle is beneficial if we are willing to learn from it.

Such a "blessing" happened to me: When I was blocked by the head of the cinema department from forming my graduate committee for my Ph.D. in Communications at The University of Southern California, I had reason to feel cheated, wronged. I had accumulated at least 74 graduate credits in communications. (I needed only 64 for my doctorate.) I was a dedicated student with top grades, especially in my area of interest, namely, creative

communications and writing. I had received enthusiastic recommendations from my professors at Temple University in Philadelphia where I
got my M.A. degree in Communications and Speech, and from the
overwhelming majority of my professors at USC in Los Angeles in the
Telecommunications and Cinema Departments -- to the point of their
recommending me for a full State scholarship.

I won that State scholarship because of their support. I lost it
because of the prejudice of one man, who, unfortunately, happened to
be the cinema department head. I have much of the dialogue of that
period documented on tape. In essence, his reason for rejecting me
was that I did not have the personality desired for graduates
representing his cinema department -- that the typical Middle Eastern
person, be he Iranian, Egyptian or Israeli -- is a "dishonest con
artist." (He knew I am a native of Israel.)

I had a long and bitter battle against the injustice of that man
and against that part of the political system of USC which condoned
it. Involved on my behalf were well-known people such as Senator
Mervyn Dymally, Jerry Lewis, Norman Taurog, Saul Lesser, even the
Anti-Defamation League...but to no avail. The department head
controlled through money power -- donations from the big film studios.
He must have felt terribly threatened by me to misuse the Police
Department and the City Attorney to harass me. To their credit, they
at last appeared to have seen through his ploy. He used any devious
means he could command -- even going so far as forgery to keep
me, finally, out.

I lost years, money, and -- most important -- ENERGY that could
have been spent in more creative, expansive areas. However, it took
this crisis to propel me to the higher level of consciousness on which
I now operate: I opened to alternatives, I mellowed, I was humbled,
and I searched and got closer to the Creator. I was steered into a
better path of EXPANDED COMMUNICATIONS rather than merely
creative communications within the "ivory tower" of intellectual
confinement. I found greater opportunity for self-expression, for
fulfillment, for creative freedom, and for helping humanity.
Consequently, one of the greatest and most cruel traumas of my life,
indeed, proved to be a great BLESSING IN DISGUISE!

Look into your own life. Pick a traumatic experience. Now
look for the blessing in disguise. Find what you have learned from it,
or could. Find what benefits you have gained or how you can
improve your life if you apply all the lessons of your painful
experience. BE PROUD OF GROWING FROM YOUR PAIN.

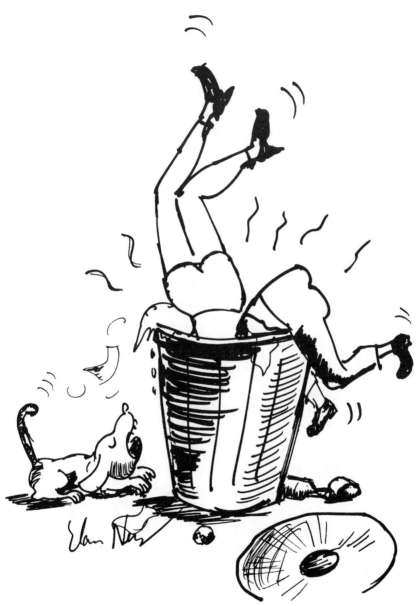

Look for the blessings in disguise,
even if the disguise is excellent!

Everybody is a teacher

Bring to mind a person who often annoys you. Stay with the first person that comes to your mind. Now tell yourself or write down the three most annoying things this person does, or simply what you dislike most about him or her. Now put yourself in the place of that person. Tell yourself the same things you dislike that you told that individual. Now, honestly examine whether the things you dislike in the other person might be things you dislike in yourself. Examine yourself as deeply as you can. Some weaknesses may be well hidden, or even dormant, lying in ambush for the right opportunity to pounce on you and take control.

THE POINT IS, WE OFTEN ATTRACT PEOPLE WHO REFLECT OUR WEAKNESSES LIKE A MIRROR. IT IS EASIER FOR US TO FIND FAULTS IN OTHERS THAN IN OURSELVES. OTHERS PROVIDE FOR US WONDERFUL OPPORTUNITIES TO EXAMINE OURSELVES.

Sometimes we are unconsciously drawn to people who irritate or hurt us, not because they necessarily reflect us, but because we need to develop some qualities such as patience or strength. These people may be unaware of being our teachers. Nonetheless, they are our teachers, appointed by life. Very likely, we are their teachers too.

Personally, I always learn from my students and clients, even the most "unfortunate and hapless" ones. I am grateful to every person in my life, including people like the department head who hurt me -- because they taught me important lessons whether they meant to or not. I am stronger, freer, and more aware because of the lessons they taught me. In turn, I hope they learn some valuable lessons from me that help with their evolution.

How to learn from your enemies

It is not easy to learn from your enemies if you are obsessed by the desire to destroy them. But, if you realize that life has provided them to teach you and to help you develop, you may look at your enemies with a curious mind and an eagerness to learn and grow. A few interesting developments may take place if you do so:

A.   You will feel a lot better. Curiosity and openness to improvement are by far more beneficial than hatred. Hatred can
destroy others, but it can also destroy you, as it is like an
acid flowing through you. It also attracts more hatred, like an
endless stream, until you are literally drowning in its poison.

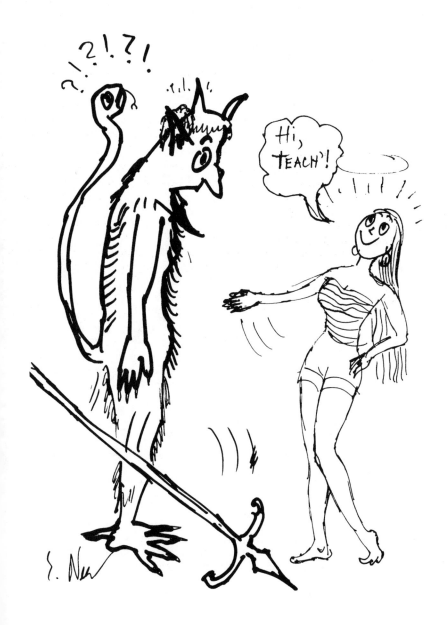

B.   As you substitute hatred toward your enemies with a quest for enlightenment, your enemies may feel less threatened and cease to threaten you. You may start a constructive dialogue that ends up with peace and love. And, in the future, your new state of consciousness may not create enemies nor attract them to you any longer.

C.   If peace with your enemies is impossible to achieve -- at least in this lifetime -- you can deal with them coolly and effectively for your own survival.

How to learn from "mistakes"

On the spiritual, Wholistic level there are no mistakes. Everything that happens to us happens for a good reason. Our state of consciousness attracts the "mistakes" we need for our growth.

I know some of you may protest, "But there are some incidents and accidents I can certainly do without. I didn't ask for, don't need and don't want these costly, painful mistakes!" Yes, I empathetically believe you. Part of you, the rational, conscious part, does not want the mistakes.   But another part, which may be totally unconscious, may produce these mistakes to teach you a lesson similar in nature to what we discussed previously in this chapter.

The thing to remember in Wholistic healing is not to brood over mistakes, but to accept them and learn the full lessons from them. When we fully accept ourselves and others, in spite of our mistakes, our self-image heightens and the flow of our love energy increases. This is definitely Wholistic healing in action! And soon there will be less need for mistakes, and fewer mistakes will be made!

Using intuition to foresee "mistakes" and avoid them

I believe our mistakes and any sufferings associated with them are only necessary as lessons, not punishment. Therefore, if we can only learn the lessons and pass the test of enlightment, we don't necessarily have to continue the suffering.

The only way I know of learning our prescribed life lessons without suffering is to expand our awareness. This will allow us a better view of the past, present, and future, helping us learn from past mistakes in order to avoid pitfalls in the present.

If you are raising a brow about expanding your awareness into the future, let me give you an illustration that will help you realize

that the task is not so "far out:" your life is like a journey. When
you get in your car to go on a trip, you have the choice of just
driving toward your destination, hoping to find it somehow, or choosing
the expanded awareness way of journeying: you get a recent map that
provides you with an accurate overview of the territory you are to
visit. You determine the route you are to take, based on what you
want to see considering the length and quality of the road in relation
to obstacles. You will choose an optimal route that will get you to
your destination in the safest, fastest, and most gas-conserving
manner.

Under certain circumstances, especially if you are a hiker, you
may find that you can increase your awareness a great deal if you
take an observation post on a mountain top, surveying in advance the
route you are going to take. Even if you don't plot a perfect plan,
your mind will be clearer from the cleaner air.

When I worked for the field intelligence of the Israel Defense
Force, we always expanded our awareness before any major military
action -- or as a preparation for a military confrontation -- through
such means as aerial photography, scouting missions, and various
intelligence reports. During a confrontation, we always kept creative
on-the-spot, minute-by-minute intelligence feedback whenever
possible, and acted according to the circumstances in the here and
now. This cumulative intelligence gathering was especially valuable
to me, as a pragmatic exercise in expanded awareness.

Similarly, in your everyday life and spiritual development,
expanded awareness will provide you with foresight that will guide
you safely toward your right path, even through perils and tribulation,
without losing sight or contact with your base from whence you
started your journey. The view ahead will provide you with purpose,
direction, and safety; the view to the rear will provide you with moral
and emotional support, balance and grounding.

When your expanded awareness "radar" detects something ahead,
your whole being will be evaluating that "something" on the basis of
previous and present ingelligence. The more aware you are, the
better your evaluation will be. It will not be limited by what you
had experienced in the past, but it will make good use of it. It will
not be biased by your hopes and visions for the future if the reality of
the here and now dictates change of course, but it will provide you
with a good balance of safety, speed, and persistence necessary for
arrival at your destination in due time and in one piece--whole!

With expanded awareness you can foresee mistakes and
obstacles (the bridge is washed out). Avoid them (find a suitable
detour). Meditate on accepting the intended lesson (patience and

moderation).   When you grow in the areas of deficiency indicated by the foreseen mistakes, you obviate the need to go through them.

By now you may ask, "How do I develop such an expanded awareness?"   That is a good question.   Just persist in studying this book with an open mind, apply what you read to everyday life, and take mind-expanding and consciousness-raising training, such as is offered by my Self-Improvement Institute.

How to prevent misfortunes in spite of feelings of impending disaster (or how a Jewish Mother worries through international channels)

Sometimes we may be hit with feelings of impending disaster. We may dream about something bad happening to us or to someone else.   We may get a warning in meditation or through other means.

We can treat such alarming visions like the unfortunate "mistakes" mentioned in the previous section of this chapter.   We can remove the trauma out of the experience by accepting in advance any experience, pleasant or unpleasant, as a constructive lesson. Even if a terrible thing has been forecast, why should we waste the good time we have now?   How "heavy" it is to live in the now with the fear of tomorrow !   And yet, there are many people whose lives are constricted by the dread of death, disease, accidents, financial loss, failure, defamation, robbery, rape, racial or religious infiltration, and political takeover.

Do you realize that by keeping the fear alive -- whether the fear is grounded or not   -- the fearers give it energy to the degree that what is feared can be materialized, or materialized sooner?

My own dear mother has been a great worrier.   In 1975, I once failed to write to her and my family in Israel for only two weeks, and she began to envision all sorts of disasters for me to the point where I started to sense the formation of destructive energies around me.   Fortunately, the negativity was relieved when my mother, in her stereotypical Jewish-motherly fashion, almost created an "international crisis" by calling up the Israeli consul in Los Angeles early in the morning to check on her 38-year-old "baby" who had survived the Israeli Army and 17 years of struggling abroad on his own. And just as a measure of added security, she had my youngest brother, Doron, call the Israeli Embassy in Washington, through the office of the Foreign Ministry in the Holy City of Jerusalem.   The upshot was that I was awakened in the wee hours of the morning from a very pleasant dream on how to save the world, with the command to immediately call Mommie and tell her I was okay.   Right then I realized my lesson that what, indeed, held me down for many years had been my mother's wondering whether I was okay. But how can you blame a Jewish mother for worrying over her firstborn baby when he deals with such "spooky" things as spiritual healing, psychokinetic energies, and the Kabala instead of becoming a medical doctor, or at least a wealthy lawyer!

But not all worrying has such an amusing end. For a few years my mother had been preoccupied with the observation that some acquaintances were developing cancer. She repeatedly and fearfully remarked: "One day I am going to catch cancer of the breast." One day she did. She materialized the vision she had nurtured with fear, and lost the breast that had nurtured me with love-milk.

About six months before my mother's cancer was medically detected, I and some other graduates of Silva Mind Control, saw a deficiency in my mother's aura (the electromagnetic field around an object). Without telling my mother about the problem so as not to give more energy to her worries and thus to the problem -- I sent her a healing cassette tape recorded especially for her. I was so confident I could help her prevent the foreseen problems from materializing. But alas! My mother sent the tape back to me with the admonition not to ever send such nonsense to her. Better I should get a "normal job," a wife, and lead an "orderly" life.

This was a case where the affected person was so attached to the vision of impending disaster that she chose to vehemently block help, practically wanting the cancer to occur (at least on the subconscious level). Had I been more advanced at the time I read disharmony in her aura, I might have helped her prevent the disaster in spite of her self-destructiveness. I would have psychically analyzed the reasons for her fear-want. If, for example, I found that she needed sympathy, attention...and that her life lesson was to be less aggressive, I would have envisioned her satisfying her needs without developing cancer, learning her lesson of relaxation and letting go without being forced into it by a horrible disease.

The concept we should understand in order to prevent imagined misfortunes is that just because we see them happen in our dreams, for instance, does not mean they must happen in life. Since all experiences are life lessons, and since a dream or a vision is also an experience -- learning the lessons from events in our minds can free us from the need to go through the events again in what we call reality. The visions may be the projection of our state of consciousness now. They are not necessarily premonitions about inescapable fate.

For example, if you dreamed that your car went off a bridge and caught on fire, destroying all its occupants, don't look forward to it happening. Perhaps the vision is symbolic, cautioning you to "drive" more carefully in your dealings with your passengers. The disaster thus will be prevented if you listen to the warning.

Or, perhaps you check the steering mechanism on your car and find it faulty. Repair it, and thank Higher Intelligence for warning you.

You may be asking now, "How do I know what the dream, vision, or premonition means and the lesson that is to be learned from it?" It is an art, sometimes perfected to almost a science. The fastest way to master it is to expand your awareness through training.

Meanwhile, there is one technique you can use which is described in the following section.

COSMIC AIKIDO: how to roll with the blow and bounce back!

Everything is energy. Pain and tension occur when energies clash, or when there is resistance. Destruction can occur during such a conflict. Damage may be averted by maneuvering the direction of the energies and their degree of focus.

Aikido is a Japanese art of self defense in harmony with the ki, or the life energy. The practitioner of Aikido can absorb the most violent blows without hurt or damage, simply by flowing with the direction of the energy. Just like a blade of grass gracefully bends until the storm is over, so does the Aikido expert. He moves smoothly with every hostile push against himself. He gets in harmony with his adversaries without losing his strength and freedom. He can swiftly rise and take control of the situation, even if pushed violently to the ground.

I have expanded the meaning of Aikido and coined the phrase "Cosmic Aikido" to encompass the application of the Aikido style of self defense Wholistically. The next time you experience conflict, ponder upon this question: which is stronger, a sheet of steel that can be arched under pressure and then regain its original shape when let go, or a piece of plate glass which is so hard it won't budge, but will shatter rather than give?

If you understand this concept, you are in touch with a powerful tool of Wholistic health on the physical, emotional, spiritual, and social levels. It can also be applied to avert foreseen problems (see preceding section). Here is how you may use it:

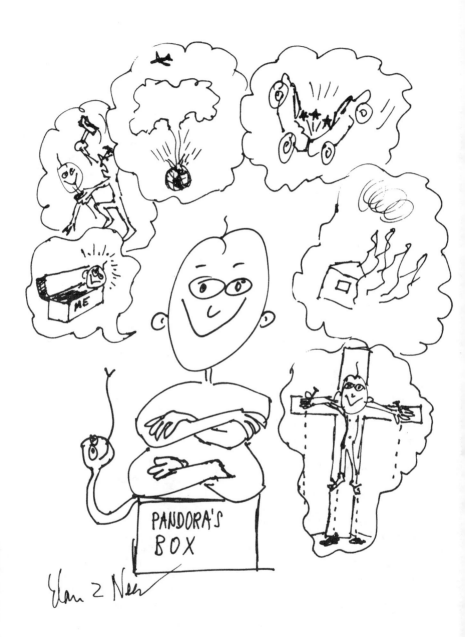

Let us go back to the vision of your car going off a bridge in a fiery crash as described in the previous section. You can use the Cosmic Aikido technique to literally edit and re-dream your vision. You apply the technique by allowing the violence of your dream to burn itself up. Instead of trying to resist the premonition of impending disaster by suppressing it (which, as in the case with pain, can unconsciously program your very destruction), flow with it, draw it out...up to a point.

See yourself getting to the bridge and starting to lose control of your car. Feel yourself prepared and accepting the almost certain disaster, praying hurriedly for enlightenment and help. Feel yourself taking in a quick but very deep breath of life, then releasing all tension and negativity out of your system, trusting and accepting that what may come is for a good reason. Let go of all fear, then see yourself barely making it to the other side of the bridge, scratchless and whole, giving thanks for your "good luck" -- promising yourself to learn all lessons that may come to you from that near disaster.

Repeat your happy ending as often as it takes until you are imbued with the conviction that you will be alright even if you may, one day, come across that hazardous bridge, literally or allegorically.

"But what if the premonition of impending disaster is so great that I cannot free myself from it?" you may ask. The more vivid your edited dream, the better your chances are to diffuse the impending disaster. Deep meditation is a most useful tool to impress all levels of consciousness with the desired positive vision. If you have not learned meditation yet and you need help fast, an expert parapsychologist or New Age teacher can guide you into effective meditation for overcoming your problem, often in one session.

Of course, developed imagination will help you in revising your "bad dream;" it, too, can be developed a great deal through meditation and mind expansion.

If you find that your revised vision is being rejected by your system as unbelievable, you must resort to a more daring maneuver of Cosmic Aikido. You may liken it to a swimmer caught in a whirlpool, threatening to swallow him. If the swimmer fights the terrifying downward pull of the water, he is bound to lose energy, get tired, and drown. But, if he courageously swims downward with the pull, he may preserve enough strength to dive into the eye of the whirlpool, out from under it, and shoot back to the surface.

As I said, this requires more courage and trust, and the ability to relax and act coolly and swiftly in the face of impending calamity. The more you learn to harmonize with the energies of life, the better you will survive its dangers.

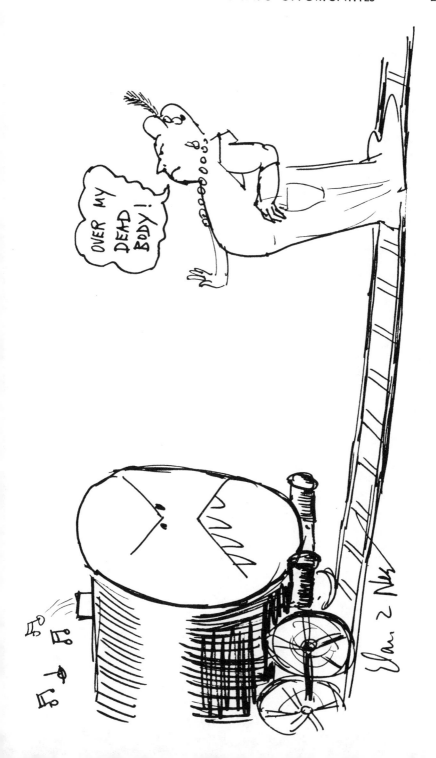

A more daring approach to the example of the car accident is to go further than wishing that you and your car come out of it scratchless. To convince your various states of consciousness to accept a less tragic ending than the crashing and burning you originally foresaw, you may have to wheel and deal with them and give in some. To dissipate more of the destructive force of the premonition of impending disaster, you may have to settle for seeing your car scratching the rail of the bridge and coming to a halt with you and your passengers getting out safely.

If the destructive energies are so strong that damaging your car is not sufficient to drain them out, you may have to go even further: see your car crashing through the rail, even catching on fire -- yet all passengers jumping out and surviving. But if you have to go that far, I would advise you seek help immediately from a competent parapsychologist.

How to use opposition to move forward
(and an interpretation of a Jewish-Christian Teacher)

Using Cosmic Aikido does not mean that you must remain a passive ball bouncing masochistically as it absorbs kicking and pounding, constantly changing shape to suit the beating. Yes, you need to absorb and roll and bounce when kicked, but nurture a mind and direction of your own. Like a ball with an integral characteristic, bounce and roll in the direction most suitable for you. You can learn to guide the energies rather than blindly submitting to them. You can have a flexible spine instead of being spineless.

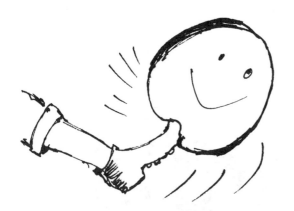
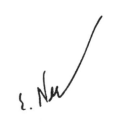

Free, unresisting and bouncy as a ball,
but KNOWING where to bounce.

The art of getting in harmony with life and experiencing Wholistic healing can enable you to use all energies, including opposing or hostile energies, for the good. When you are able to flow with and channel your energies, you will become like a sailboat that happily and effortlessly travels the rough but beautiful sea of life by using all winds -- including opposing ones -- to propel itself forward toward its destination: a paradise island of peace and light.

Next time you experience an opposition, try not to stiffen up angrily or fearfully. Humbly turn with the opposing force. Keep on turning, effortlessly using the opposing energy to turn and carry you toward your desired destination. It occurred to me that this is basically what the Jewish-Christian Master Jesus meant when he preached about turning the other cheek.

As you develop your sense of rhythm and movement of life through expanding your awareness, the turning, bending and focusing of energies will become easier and easier, until living will be transformed into a cosmic dance of fulfillment.

Meditations and Affirmations for turning problems into opportunities

Relax. Get into your pyramid of white light inside the Oval Love Energy Transceiver of Self-Improvement as described at the end of Chapter 1. Get to the point in the meditation where you experience the white beam of cosmic light inside your center. Now tell yourself through your center: "I realize every problem is an opportunity for growth. I don't waste any problem by trying to suppress it. I face it courageously. I ask what lesson it has for me. I am not afraid of problems any more. I know that by learning from my difficulties, I will have fewer and fewer problems. With every failure, small or big, I grow. With every obstacle, I get stronger. I learn from my enemies too. Every day and in every way I get stronger and better. Yet, I am flexible and free. I can flow with the punches. I can fall and rise again. And my trust in the goodness and fulfillment of my mission in life is growing stronger with every experience, unpleasant or pleasant. Every moment brings me another experience, every relationship is learning. I welcome all learning and am expanding my awareness all the time. I am motivated to experience more fully, to live more completely. I accept life. I love life. I flow with life. Day by day and in every way, I am getting better and better at using all of life's energies constructively and creatively for the good."

Visualize now, or think about, three problems in your life in the order that they come to you. Ask yourself what lessons they offer and what blessings may be in disguise. Imagine yourself applying these lessons. In your mind go over your day, face each problem and ask for the lesson. Then release any anxiety, even if the lesson has not surfaced to your conscious mind. Just know it will come in due time.

The best time for this meditation is at the end of the day. By doing it, or including it in your regular meditation -- perhaps with the help of a tape recorder -- you will have a calmer night. And while you are asleep you may be further learning your lessons and incubating creative solutions to problems.

CHAPTER 3

HEALING PAIN:
PHYSICAL, EMOTIONAL, AND FINANCIAL. . .
AND SOME DANGERS!

The danger in healing too soon

Since every experience, including pain, is a lesson that must be learned well, an incomplete experience is an incomplete lesson that must be repeated.

It is possible to "heal" too soon, that is, before the lesson is fully learned. A healing may appear to take place. The symptoms such as pain and discomfort associated with the disease may be suppressed or even alleviated. When this occurs, the pressure to do something about the disease disappears. However, the disease, or at least its roots, may be stealthily harboring another attack.

Unfortunately, many ailments are treated with the emphasis on curing the symptoms. Whether the help given is through conventional medicine or through spiritual treatment, if the manifest and painful part of the disease is cut out, but the live roots remain below, the patient is not fully cured. In fact, too early a "healing" may cause complacency and neglect of something serious. To heal Wholistically, one must become whole. One cannot Wholistically heal one problem at the expense of another. The purpose of healing, thus, should be the whole person: mind, soul, and body in harmony. And the best preventive medicine should be, accordingly, keeping in harmony within and without.

Do not kill your friend, the pain

When a sufferer of a physical or emotional pain demands from me an instant cure of the pain, I usually do the following:

A.   I remind the sufferer that I may not and do not practice medicine, since I am not a medical doctor. For medical treatment, I advise the sufferer to seek a competent physician.

B.   I remind the sufferer that the only healing I strive toward is the healing he brings about from within.

C.   I request the sufferer to carefully read and sign a release form clearly putting the responsibility on his own shoulders.

D.   I collect a payment for my TIME -- not healing -- in advance. This I have found is necessary not only to enable me to continue to devote all my time to helping people, but also to re-affirm the sufferer's trust and openness so important in Wholistic healing.

E.   I advise the sufferer that even though he or she may have witnessed instantaneous relief from pain by some of my audience or students during my lectures, seminars, or religious services, or heard of a "miraculous" healing during my private sessions, I guarantee nothing. I am only an instrument. The healing process is between Nature and the sufferer.

F.   I tell the sufferer I will not encourage or be part of using spiritual and psychic healing as an opium to drug the suffering. I will try to help with the pain only to the extent it is necessary for the sufferer to be able to concentrate during the session. I will strive to help the sufferer to deal with the CAUSES of the pain, so that if the sufferer is ready and willing to learn the necessary lesson, this pain will spontaneously and permanently vanish.

This last part is most important. I do not seek clients and students who would forever depend on me or my techniques for alleviation from pain. My mission is to teach that only we develop our pain or let go of it, depending upon our own evolvement and willingness to assume responsibility and take charge. Working on the pain alone can only temporarily alleviate it, creating greater and greater dependency on the "curing" drug or even the spiritual, meditative, or hypnotic technique. Or it may "cure" one pain and cause other pains to erupt instead. (For a more complete picture, review the first part of Chapter 2.)

If I help a sufferer of an acute and repeated headache to "get rid" of the pain through some of the instant, superficial, psychic techniques available, without going into the cause of the pain, I may be helping the sufferer to camoflage a budding tumor. The pain is there not to punish, but to help -- not to torture, but to warn. Therefore, one of the important skills required for Wholistic healing is to listen. So let us listen to our pain. It IS our friend!

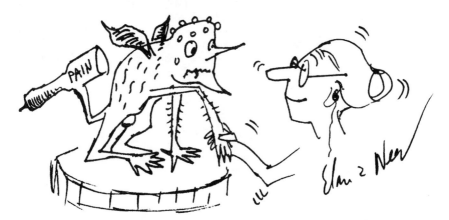

Getting acquainted with your pain

Getting pain, as you know, is easy. But really getting to know your pain is not.

What do I mean by getting to know your pain? I mean listening to what it says. Looking it right in the face. Accepting it!

Don't we know our pain the second we feel it? Often not. Often we begin to sense it, physically or emotionally, and immediately and frantically we try to kill it, or turn our backs on it, or run, run, run.... Most of us have developed such a strong habit of trying to drown our pain with pleasures that our constant attempt at avoiding and evading pain has become a conditioned reflex: headache, upset stomach, sleeplessness? Automatically the hands reach to the pill, to kill, to kill, to kill.... And kill it does: the human organism, the natural biochemical balance, the personality, the mind. Sometimes a slow death, sometimes a fast one.

But the pain cannot be killed that way, at least not so long as the body lives...and spiritually speaking, not even after the body has been demolished. The soul will continue to suffer until it learns from the pain the full, intended lesson. At most, the pain may be temporarily knocked out. So next time that we reach for the pill, or the cigaret, or the alcohol, or the addictive fattening food, let us remember: knowing our pain in depth is the only sure way to say goodbye to it.

What about "harmless" ways to avoid or forget pain, such as buying a new hat, indulging sexually, changing location? First, these ways may not be so harmless if done for the wrong reason. Second, let us once and for all stop seeking ways of not facing our pain. STOP RIGHT NOW! Catch your breath. Inhale deeply, and release...all fears of the unknown, all fears of hurt. Look at your pain. LOOK AT YOUR PAIN NOW! It is not after you to destroy you. It is your friend. It is only here to tell you something for your own good. You had better listen before life catches you by the throat, hits you right on your head, cracking your mind wide open, striking you with such mental or physical anguish that you will cry out, "I will listen! I will listen! Just tell me what to do and how to change. Hurry. I can't take it any more!"

I am channeling and writing for you with love. A true love. Unconditional love. Not to please. Not to possess. Just to express and share and care. I allow my passion to flow through to you as I am shouting and repeating my message over and over again! Better let the torrent and intensity of my words penetrate your shield of insecurity, than wait till the pain builds up to a devastating explosion.

Being especially obstinate and stoic in resistance, it took the powerful emotional blow of losing my wife and children before I just began to get acquainted with my pain and its message of life.   For years I had been faced with events which I did not let touch my emotions.   I had friends who were killed in service, but I was a "strong and virile male" who would not be caught dead with a tear in his eyes.   I needed a powerful blow to penetrate my thick intellectual shell.   In the beginning I felt I had to turn my boy's and girl's pictures to the wall so I wouldn't see their beautiful images and painfully miss them.   But then, something within me said that I should face their pictures, get in touch with my feelings, and release them.

So I followed my inner guidance and put my children's photos in every room in order to see them wherever I went in my apartment. For two weeks the photos seemed to torture my soul with the memory of my Tamir and Shalva, my boy and girl.   And I was also seized with a severe physical pain in my chest and throat.   But I kept looking at my Tamir and Shalva, remembering vividly the long hours we spent together, the dirty diapers I often changed, the bloody head, the tears, the laughter, the Bible stories I told them, the hikes, the swimming and music lessons I gave them, the fooling around and roughing it up on the floor, the hugs and kisses, and their beautiful squeals of joy, "Aba, Aba"! (meaning "father, father"! in Hebrew) with which they greeted me as they hopped into my arms when I would return from work.

And then, suddenly, after years of suppressed tears, my eyes started flowing.   I let go and sobbed on and off for days.   And the pain on my heart and in my throat was washed away with the flood of my tears.   All of a sudden I could look at my kids' beloved faces and be aware of no more pain.   What a feeling of freedom!

But I guess I was healed too soon from my pain.   I was always too good at getting rid of pain and discomfort too fast.   I did not open wide enough.   I closed up again, learning only part of my lesson.   So I deserved another blow.   And the trouble I attracted to me at USC (see "Unveiling the blessings in disguise" in Chapter 2) seemed to be an additional, sufficiently penetrating lesson to keep me open and cleansed -- able to continually mature emotionally and spiritually.

These have been some of my rewards for getting to know my pain. If you have not yet reaped rewards from your pain -- if you want to reduce pain, read on!

A simple technique to alleviate pain without drugs or meditation

It is simple. You just have to get acquainted with your pain a bit better.

Wherever you are, just focus your full attention on your pain. Describe it in detail, ceaselessly, as it is NOW. Keep on describing it, even if you bore yourself and your friends. Repeat the description if there is no change. Don't look back. Don't be held by past experience with your pain or your expectation for the future. It does not matter now what the habitual patterns of your pain are. Free yourself from the addiction to any such habit pattern. DESCRIBE YOUR PAIN NOW. Be as graphic as possible. Even use your imagination.

Ask yourself how deep the pain is (is it on the surface, or is it an inch below your skin?). What shape does it have? Describe it with your hands as if you are touching an object in front of you. Draw it on paper or in the air, if you wish. But keep on describing it. Keep on moving forward. What color does your pain seem to have? Use your imagination and guess a color or colors even if you don't seem to see a thing. (Incidentally, you are developing your sensitivity and psychic powers now.) Feel and describe the quality of pain. Is it sharp or dull? Does it pulsate? Show the rhythm of the pulsation.

Don't let the pain out of your sight for a second. Even if it moves, or spreads, or changes -- keep following it with your expanding awareness. Smell it, if you can. Guess the smell if need be. Does your pain make sounds? What kind of sounds? Groaning, swishing, pounding, clicking, grinding, crackling, whistling, thundering? Is it a metallic sound? Or is it like paper or bones or wood? Don't limit yourself by my questions and choices of answers. Follow your own feelings.

Don't be surprised if, after a few minutes of industrious description, you find no more to describe. You see, by describing your pain, you force yourself to pay attention to it and learn to know it intimately. While you do so, you accept your pain instead of fighting it. Tension, then, goes...and the pain often goes with it.

A meditative psychic technique to deal with pain

I'll reveal to you an effective technique which some other New Age teachers and I use in our courses. I did, however, make some improvement in the technique.

Bring yourself into a meditative state inside your pyramid of light as described at the end of Chapter 1. Now, imagine a cloud-like chair or bed in your pyramid. Sit or lie there comfortably with the back of your head to the north and feet to the south. Beside you is a switch. Turn the switch on and imagine seeing a split white movie screen coming down in front of you and above. It has an ugly brown frame and a sign: Pain Communications. Even though your pain is your teacher, the ugly brown frame will remind you that you will see the pain for learning purposes only, not to program it into unnecessary continuance.

On the left side of the split screen you will later project the image of your pain as inspired by your higher self or superconsciousness. On the right side, you will later project the image of your pain as you perceive it (similarly to what you did in the previous section).

Get ready now for the left side of the split screen. At the count of three, you will turn another switch and your superconsciousness will instantaneously project your main pain (or the pain of another person you wish to help) on the left side of the split screen. Don't intellectualize the way the pain would look. It may surprise you with some important insight as to its nature and causes if you just let the pain spontaneously flash on the screen. It is likely to appear symbolically as in a dream, or it may even assume a human form or an x-ray-like "scientific" picture of an afflicted organ. Remember, nothing is going to scare you. You are totally protected. One, two, three! Project the pain!

Let the pain remain on the screen, stationary or animated. Get whatever first impressions of it come to you. Then focus on the right side of the split screen. At the count of three you will turn on another switch and deliberately project the pain the way you can rationally describe it as you feel it (or if it is someone else', as you guess it to be). You may use your imagination, but project -- or even paint or sculpture -- the pain exactly as you sense it right now. Even if the pain is emotional, project it on the screen. If you have to use your imagination to draw an abstract picture of the pain and its movement and rhythm, do so. One, two, three!

Look now at the two sides of the split screen at once. Compare the two images of the same pain and draw your conclusions.

Now, at the count of three, turn a third switch on to merge the two screens. One, two, three! Look at the merged, or expanded image of the pain. Does it mean anything to you? Do you get any clue about the cause of the pain and what lesson there is to learn? Talk to the pain, vocally or in your mind. Ask it why it is there. What message does it bear. What should be done to graduate from the lesson so that there will be no more need for the pain. If the pain reminds you of someone but you don't know who, ask it to remove its mask. You may remove as many masks as you feel necessary. At all times treat the pain with respect, even if it should look horrible. Fear not. Remember that pain is a teacher, even if a cruel one. Thank the pain for its cooperation, and politely send it away. When the split screen of pain communications is clear, turn the appropriate switch to lift the screen back into the ceiling.

In my Wholistic Oneness Self-Improvement Training, we go into finer detail in analyzing and healing pain; but for a technique divulged through the printed word, this should suffice. It should help you a great deal if you do not hesitate to "play along" with it, rather than dismiss it with your "adult" intellectual mind. Always bring yourself back in due time with the suggestion that you return to the objective world at the time you pre-set or whenever it is safe and good to do so, with the affirmation that you will feel and be better than before -- wide awake, full of vitality and joy, and in harmony with life.

Dealing with "financial pain" and an illustration good for any pain

If the pain you are dealing with is more abstract than physical pain, if you suffer because of financial difficulties, for example, the same meditative psychic technique can be used. Naturally, you may need more imagination and inspiration here, but it still works.

A salesman was taking my Wholistic Oneness Self-Improvement training with the goal of making more money. His superconsciousness projected on the left side of the split screen, to his complete surprise, his beloved mother whom he had not seen for a long time. His financial pain was depicted as his mother!

Before he even had a chance to scratch his head (not recommended during meditation) or even ask the symbolic image of his mother for more explanation, the realization flashed in his head that his mother was very tight with money. The realization that followed immediately was that her holding on so tightly to money affected his attitude toward money and was restricting the flow of money through him.

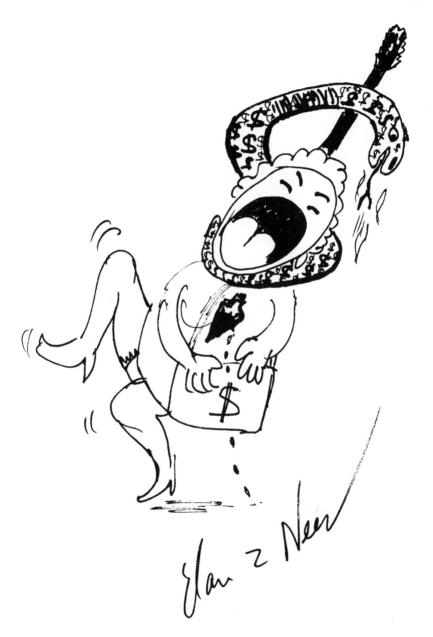

The salesman thus already received a diagnosis and prescription from his Higher Self, obviating the need to go any further with the mechanics of the technique, or even to the right side of the split screen. He knew now that he must work on letting money flow through him freely, rather than holding onto it tightly and fearfully while expecting his customers to have the same tight attitude toward money that his mother had.

Since he experienced an immediate change in consciousness, his financial pain in the image of his mother vanished from the screen. There was no more need for the pain that was caused by his attachment to money and the belief that everyone is attached to money, making transactions difficult. During the training he was able to "let go" in general and release his mother in particular. Within three months the salesman's volume had skyrocketed. As a nice "fringe benefit," it was reported that his love life was also phenomenally improved and that he was glowing with self-assuredness, enthusiasm, and wholesome magnetism!

So you see, you don't have to artificially bind yourself by the technique. Flow with it. It does not have to be so intricate as it may first appear. Improvise on it. Do what feels right to you. At Self-Improvement Institute, we repeatedly stress the importance of self-reliance and independence, even from our teachings or techniques, as soon as possible. It is your mind and life you are dealing with, even if you are trying to help another person. It is your responsibility to take good care.

A parapsychological technique to release pain-causing tension

(Or how an advertising executive freed himself through the telephone from a headache and a pain in the neck)

Here is a parapsychological technique which I developed while helping some students and clients deal with their pain. You may use it in or out of a meditative state of mind. I find it very effective even without going into an altered state of consciousness.

I will give you an actual example of how I used this technique over the telephone on a graduate of my training, a top advertising executive:

He complained about an excruciating tension pain in the back of his head and neck. I went with him through the basic pain-awareness technique described in this chapter under "A simple technique to alleviate pain...." Consequently, his pain shrank to the size of a fist in the back of his neck. The pain lodged there and seemed quite stubborn. The executive had an important meeting to attend and we agreed it was urgent to relieve the pain. To do so within the few minutes we both had available, we resorted to a swift use of the imagination.

I told him to pretend to take the fist-like pain in his hand. He was now observing and feeling its painful pulsations. Then both of us -- I through my ESP, and he more directly through his imagination -- focused an orange light from our third eyes in our foreheads onto the fist-like pain. We were willing and visualizing the orange ray to permeate the "fist" with loving, freeing, relaxing energy.

Then we placed the "fist" on the advertising executive's desk. As the fist-like pain was being bathed in liberating, loosening orange light, the executive and I were discussing the tensions of the day. Coming as no surprise was the observation by the executive that one of his secretaries was "a pain in the neck." She was the most experienced and fastest, but very temperamental and "unapproachable."

After arriving at the conclusion that no human being, however "indispensable", is worth such pain, he resolved to face her with constructive criticism without delay, despite her moodiness.

By now the fist was aglow with orange light and was somewhat looser and bigger. But the pain was still very much there. Now it looked like a big knot. So, of course, we proceeded to untie the knot. As that respectable executive was fooling around like a child with the fantasized knot on his desk, suddenly he realized that there was nothing more to untie. The "fist" had vanished and so did the pain in his neck !

And, by the way, if you think that secretary was fired and replaced with a sweet young thing, you are wrong. She respects her boss more for his openness, and she is working with my mind-expanding methods on solving her personal problems. I also understand she is due for a big bonus next Christmas. But this is another fun story to be told another time !

Rising above pain through expanded awareness

(Getting into the swing of life, between the polarities, without suffering)

It is the natural rhythm of life to pulsate. Everything seems to pulsate: our hearts, our moods, the cycles of day and night, the

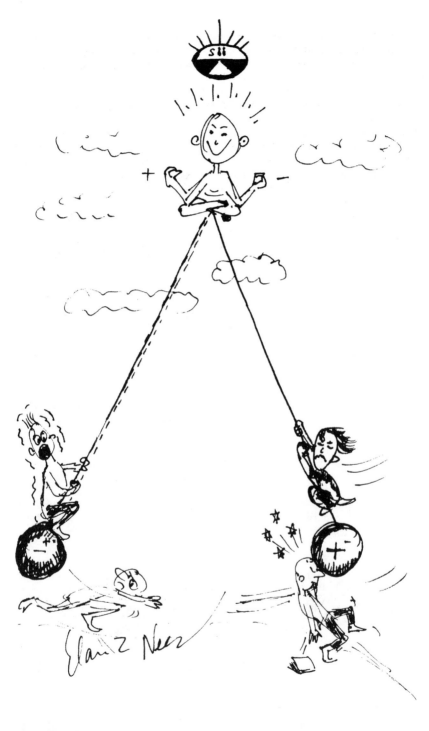

seasons.... Everything seems to swing between tension and relaxation, contraction and expansion, agony and ecstasy, low and high, thin and wide, hard and soft, cold and hot, hate and love, minus and plus, negative and positive.

We are constantly fluctuating between the extremes of the opposite polarities. The secret of harmony with life and Wholistic health is not fighting the swing of life, but joining it. It is the fighting that causes most pain, disease, and failure.

How can we master life instead of painfully being subjected to its changeability ? The answer appears paradoxical and requires special training. We must discipline ourselves to swing to the celestial music of life without swinging.

Let me explain this very crucial concept of harmony. It is our bodies and ego-dominated personalities that give us pain when they develop disharmony with the pulsations of life. It is our bodies and personalities that suffer when we attempt to resist change, e.g., not accepting natural maturity, or blindly holding onto bygone realities and habits. If we are pushed forward (and life is pushing whether we want it to nor not), but keep our sights only backward, we are bound to have a devastating collision. This will also occur if we try to block the change of others, e.g., parents interfering with their New Age children.

The ultra-religious parents of one of my graduates suffered immeasurably because they would not accept the fact that their over-30-year-old daughter was old enough to date whomever she wished, and to come home even after 10:00 p.m. They constantly expressed their frustrations to such a degree that they called her a whore in front of the entire neighborhood, no matter how innocent their daughter was. They even threatened her with a knife when she refused to rush into matrimony with a neurotic man they picked for her on the strength of his superficial financial and ritual qualities.

When our maladjusted mental attitude is transferred to our bodies, we may cause aches, diseases and deformities. Even cancer may be traced to cells resisting change, or changing against the rhythm and trend of life. Research indicates that women brought up with the belief that enjoying sex is sinful -- from the devil -- are prone to develop "devilish" cancer in their female organs. Even sex hallowed by the security of marriage does not seem to protect them from the "evil" in their contaminated minds . Because the moment they derive pleasure from intercourse with their husbands -- pleasure being the natural accompanying sensation -- the "evil" in their minds is turned on their "sinning" bodies, causing anything from frigidity to cancer.

On the other hand, we do not want to swing and sway aimlessly with every fad, with every fly-by-night idea, with every whim, with every impulse. We want a measure of solidity and stability. We want to cherish some principles of morality and good conduct, some traditions of the glories and lessons of the past, some guidelines of the sages and saints of our religions and philosophies.

But how do we strike a happy balance? How do we swing with the pendulum of life without suffering extreme, violent changes? How do we avoid having our heads smashed by the impersonal, powerful pendulum?

There is only one way I know of: expanded awareness, expanded centeredness, higher consciousness -- ENLIGHTENMENT.

Let me illustrate graphically. Look at the cartoon drawing of the swinging pendulum. Note that as we rise on it, our awareness becomes more expanded and our swinging becomes less extreme. In fact, I developed a formula to this effect:

$$\text{Degree of Harmony} = \frac{\text{Height of Awareness}}{\text{Extreme of Swing}}$$

So, in order to improve our degree of harmony, we must raise our awareness. When we do so, we acquire a wider view of the swing of the pendulum of life. This wider view, this expanded awareness, allows us to experience the swinging to its extremes without being emotionally engrossed in it. Ego and fear-motivated emotional entanglements restrict our freedom and awareness, muddy our thinking. When we are violently and haplessly being pushed by the pendulum from one extreme to the other, our awareness is down there below at the end of the string -- at the weight -- where there is most friction and danger of collision. When we are at that low level of awareness, we are prone to suffer the full weight of the mighty pendulum , and to be pushed from one crisis to another without understanding what is happening to us.

Once we realize there may be more to life than uncontrollable crises, we begin seeking the path. Many of us may need to be humbled and cracked open by "heavy experiences" before we begin searching for a better way. A few are "lucky" enough to see the light before our hurt is too great.

As we seek for a better way, our consciousness rises on the string holding the pendulum. Pretty soon we can be "up there" on the string of consciousness, having a full view to the right and the left and all around. We can foresee where the pendulum will go, and we can see clearly whence it came. Our here and now awareness encompasses wider and wider scopes of the relative time of the past through the future. Nothing then shocks us or knocks us off balance.

Through our expanded awareness we know it all and are part of it all. When we foresee trouble and pain, we also are one with the peace and joy of the past and are sustained and inspired by it.

When we reach the apex of awareness, we become masters. We are then on top, one with the source of the "triangle" of the swinging pendulum. We then enjoy a full view of life, experience with our awareness any point within the scope of life -- any or all points simultaneously -- and yet maintain our peaceful, centered, trauma-free observation point. When we are there, we are on top of the world. We do not have, then, to physically and emotionally go through suffering. We can learn by viewing. We know the lessons of life through our Wholistic awareness.

Hypnotic and self-hypnotic technique for total relaxation

Bring yourself into your Love Energy Transceiver of Self-Improvement as described at the end of Chapter 1. Imagine that you can see your own brain. It is pulsating in harmony with the universal rhythm of life. It is aglow with liberating, healing orange light. At the count of three it will reproduce the Love Energy Transceiver of Self-Improvement inside your brain. One, two, three!

The orange oval shape with its seven rays and the white pyramid within is sending a message of blessing and relaxation through your brain and throughout your nervous system to your entire being. With the power of your mind, direct your Love Energy Transceiver of Self-Improvement down your central nervous system. Perceive it crawling down your neck toward your spine, massaging and relaxing your nerves and muscles. Perceive it coming down your spine, vertabra by vertabra loving you, centering you, freeing you, relaxing every fiber in your body, mind, and soul. Feel it traveling down to your tail bone and slowly up again. Follow it back to your brain. Feel charged with cosmic energy of relaxing, freeing love-light.

From your Love Energy Transceiver of Self-Improvement and through your nervous system, broadcast the following message to your whole being: "Relax, harmonize, be whole.... I am in effortless control of my entire system. I accept my entire self with love, so I let myself be. I let go of guilt, anger, fear and tension. I let go of addictions and all toxins of mind, body and soul. As I let go I expand and open. I open myself with trust to Higher Intelligence. I let the Great Life Force flow through me unhindered. As I feel the loving cosmic energies glow through my being, I allow all my levels of consciousness to absorb and digest all lessons my pain has taught me.

I even allow my pain's lessons into my cell consciousness without the need for intellectual comprehension. I, therefore, allow for learning on any level so I can be released from my pain, emotional or physical, in due time -- now or whenever I am ready.

I let go of my fear of pain. I let go of blockages to learning. I let go of my armor. I am free and protected. I need no shield. I become even better protected, even stronger and freer as I learn the lessons from my experiences. I relax, I let go. I am free. I am free to learn. I am free to feel. I am free to express. I am free of pain.

I will wake up in due time, at a pre-set hour, or whenever it is safe and important for my total well-being, calm, relaxed, yet revitalized and flowing with the joy of life.

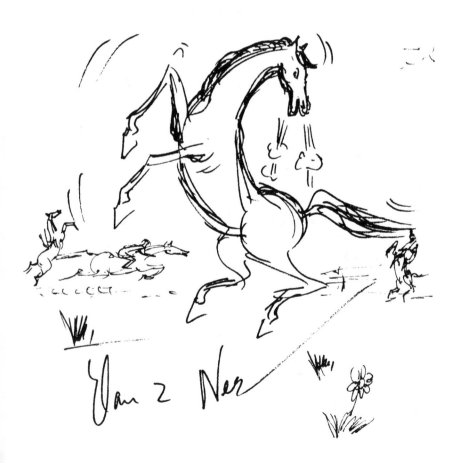

CHAPTER 4

HEALING DISEASE THE SAFE, NATURAL WAY

Everyone can heal himself or others

Often people look upon a psychic healer as a very special person. Indeed, we are all very special people: you and I, he and she.

At my Self-Improvement Institute one of my greatest challenges is NOT to let my students and clients develop any kind of dependency upon me. I remind them over and over again that I cannot do any- thing for them except inspire self-realization. I can, perhaps, teach them about something, but as illustrated in Chapter 1 under the section "Communication Problems...", the whole learning is done from within the individual by acting and reacting on one's own.

The New Age way is for each individual to become a clear channel of Universal Knowledge through his/her own center. New Age clear individuals can still seek the counsel of their teachers, live or dead. They can still respect the words of their gurus, psychiatrists, physicians, priests, ministers, rabbis, etc. But they would use them as inspiration and enlightenment, not as crutches. There are good teachers and bad teachers, true leaders and false leaders. The only way to find the true path for yourself is to maintain your own center within, through which you are linked to the Infinite Knowledge and the Universal Consciousness.

When you achieve such EXPANDED CENTEREDNESS...even if only to a certain degree and even if only occasionally, such as through prayer and meditation -- you realize that only you can heal yourself. By taking responsibility for your own decisions, you realize that even when a miracle cure is administered to you by the greatest physician, it is you -- consciously or not -- who allows the healing to take place. As far as this phenomenon is concerned, THERE IS ONLY SELF-HEALING.

When you are enlightened, you become confident and centered. Then you do not have to lean on the authority of a person outside of you to inspire you to allow the self-healing to take place. Through your center you can then inspire yourself to self-heal. And when you allow for such inspiration, your confidence and light can contagiously illuminate less confident people to heal themselves. Thus, you become a healer too!

Just as we can transfer disease of body and mind to weaker or unillumined persons, we can also share our wholeness and positiveness.

But how do we become confident enough to heal ourselves and contagiously heal others? By letting go and allowing Nature to work her "miracles"!

The secret of letting go

This is probably the most important "secret" of Wholistic healing: letting go. It is the simplest "secret," yet for many of us it is one of the most difficult to practice.

Why is letting go so important? Because by healing ourselves or helping others heal themselves, we simply let the healing take place. You see, our "healing powers" are really only our ability to let the Great Life Force flow through us unhindered. It is the Life Force that is the real healer!

Our great task, therefore, is to learn not to interfere with this natural and spontaneous healing force. And interfere we do: with our attachments, addictions, insecurities, egos, intellects, and unnatural foods and drugs.

The importance of emotional clearance

The paths of life are littered with blocks. But most of the blocks we encounter on the outside are recreations of the mental blocks within. If we believe we are weak and sickly, this is what life will produce for us. If we believe everybody is out to get us and that we are doomed to failure, no matter how many opportunities may be out there for us, we will manage to collide with the only tree along the wide and free path. We will recreate in reality the failure we created psychologically.

The fastest, most sensible way to clear our paths to peace, prosperity and wholeness is to clear out inner paths. Think how wonderful it could be if we could simply sit in the privacy of our rooms and widen roads on a street map, design bridges, shorten roads, remove obstacles, and then just know that our reality has changed to suit our revised and improved map!

WE CAN DO SUCH MAPPING IN THE PRIVACY OF OUR MINDS; REALITY WILL START TRANSFORMING ACCORDINGLY!

But how do we remove mental blocks? The older we are, the longer we tend to hold onto our emotional hang-ups. The longer we are attached to a problem, the more entangled in it we may become, and the harder it could be to release it. Yet, emotional clearance is a must if we are to allow for life's energies to work for us and through us.

Let us compare our human vehicle of energies -- our minds and bodies -- to a magnifying glass. If the magnifying glass is dirty and poorly shaped, or if it is cracked, the rays of the sun will be misdirected and diffused through it and could not ignite a fire. Also, an image of an object through the glass would look distorted rather than magnified and clear.

Conversely, if the magnifying glass is clean, polished, well ground and whole, it will focus even mild sun rays with such intensity that it could start a fire. Objects would look larger and clearer through it to the minutest details.

To get an undistorted view of life, to magnify our awareness, to be able to focus our energies on an obstacle and burn a hole in it, or to focus on a goal and realize it, we must be polished by life, clear in our thinking, grounded and centered with our emotions.

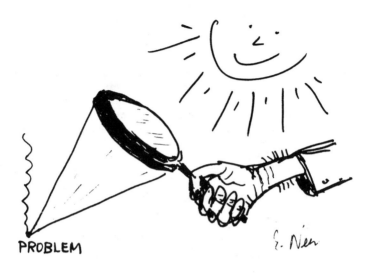

PROBLEM

To effectively focus energies on problem solving and goal realization, we must be clear, polished, and grounded. It is in our hands!

A technique of releasing and removing feelings of guilt, fear and anger

Here is a common and effective technique for release and emotional clearance: prepare three lists. One list should mention briefly all of the traumatic or painful events in your life, going back from the present to the past. The second list should include all people who angered you or hurt you. The third list should include all people you hurt, angered, or whom you feel guilty toward.

You need not go into detail. Even if you don't remember the exact name or details of an event, list any person or event that at any time was associated in your mind with negative feelings. Even people whom you may love 99% of the time, if there was or is the slightest displeasure with them, they should be included. Better to include over-lapping people and events than to leave one emotional block stone unturned!

Keep these lists prominently displayed or easily available to you. Keep adding people and events to them as you need to release anger, guilt, or any other feelings of anxiety towards them, including attachment. Include even dead people, such as a deceased husband, even if you had a marvelous relationship -- if there might be but the slightest bit of bitterness about "why did he leave me?"

Every day, at least once before you retire, look at the lists. Briefly review them, and tell the people and events, out loud or in your mind: "I release you. I release you. I accept you as you are or as you were. I thank you for all the lessons of life you gave me whether you intended to give them or not. I accept myself for giving you the lessons of life necessary for you. I free you (or, forgive you if it feels right) and free myself (and/or forgive myself). I remove all possible blocks connected with you from my life. Life flows freely through me now. And so it is."

Now wash your feet in cold water (and if you can stand it, your entire body), knowing you will continue to release blocks through the nerve endings in your feet while asleep.

Go to bed, and in a meditative state, rapidly review the entire three lists and release, release, release....

Freeing yourself and others from constricting and sickening ties ("real" ones or in your mind)

A recently divorced young lady came to me for help. She had a very painful swollen stomach that was not evacuated for five days, and which no drug or enema could relieve. As a last resort, before she was to subject herself to harsh emergency treatment in a hospital, she decided to try my natural approach to relief.

I guided her through meditation to get in touch with all the constricting feelings within her. Inspired by psychic communications with the people in her life who played a part in her personal drama, she learned her lessons from them and released them.

Following it, she received the suggestion that as soon as she completed digesting and integrating the lessons, she would feel that the constriction in her bowels -- an actual hard and painful block -- would have no more reason to exist. Before the night was over, she would go to the toilet and painlessly evacuate the accumulative physical and psychological excrement.

A half hour later she had a total cleansing of her bowels and soul, and she reported to me that she felt as if she were born again!

You can do similar things for yourself, bringing to mind the people with whom you may be entangled through hate, guilt, fear or sorrow...learn your lessons from them, and release them as described in the previous sub-chapter.

Focus, subsequently, on your ailment, and suggest to yourself that with any release or discharge of any kind, you permanently free yourself from these people as you free them from yourself, without malice.

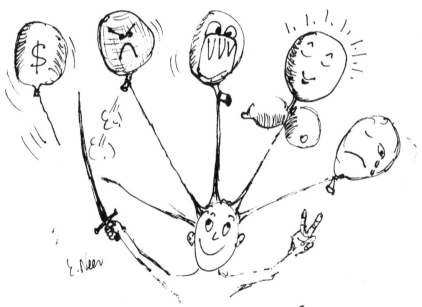

LIST HERE YOUR TIES

The question of forgiving versus releasing those who wronged you

Many religious leaders preach forgiveness. I don't choose to dissipate much energy on an academic debate concerning semantics.

I do believe that "forgiving" to most people means taking for granted that the forgiven is guilty of wrongdoing. This may lead to a patronizing attitude that can interfere with truly learning the lesson from the "forgiven" person.

What I suggest is that you do not concern yourself with forgiving those who wronged you (or those you think wronged you). Instead, just release them with thanks for your lesson and growth. Of course, if your religious belief demands you forgive and that you may be damaged by guilt if you don't, forgive. If, however, you find it impossible to forgive certain people, then just release them as I suggested. You cannot afford to hold grudges -- grudges are poisonous.

Things to do to release toxins out of your system

In addition to the methods described before, there is a simple way to release your entire system: Expand all your natural functions. Every time you relieve yourself in the bathroom, hold the index, middle finger and thumb of one hand together if you can -- for harmony and unity of soul, mind and body -- and tell yourself: "I am thoroughly cleansing my mind, soul and body from all toxins."

If you have had a special physical, emotional, or financial problem you want to release, bring it to mind and consciously release it as you naturally cleanse your system. You can even use this technique on behalf of someone you want to help. Then envision that person relieved and well.

Any other function of release can be used to increase the cleansing powers of our bodies and to effect cleansing of the mind and conditions as well. Do not miss an opportunity: if you sneeze, release; if you shout, release; if you perspire, clear your throat, spit, sob, burp, pass wind, climax, ejaculate, or even squeeze a pimple -- release....

Another releasing routine I recommend that you use by itself, or to reinforce the other methods, is to wash your feet in cold water before going to bed. In addition to enjoying sparkling clean and freshly smelling feet (which at least your bedmate, if any, would appreciate), the nerve endings of your entire body will be stimulated.

As you fall asleep, just know you are releasing all impurities of mind, soul and body through your feet, and will keep on releasing them even while asleep.

If you wish me to share my personal version of this cold treatment with you, just tune in to my shower late at night, and often early in the morning as well. The blood chilling screams you'll hear are mine, as I give myself the hot-cold-hot-cold-hot-cold...shower. This is almost as good a release as sex and, in addition, it keeps my circulation vigorous and my skin immune to cold. It also improves my vocal cords, scares away evil spirits, and teaches tolerance to my neighbors.

Finding the cause of the cause of the cause of the malady...
(or do you need to find it?)

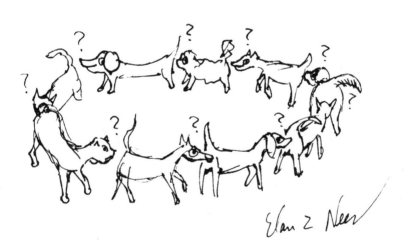

Elan Z Neev

Everything is an unbroken chain of cause and effect. If we attack one problem alone which is most likely only a symptom, without taking into consideration the total picture, we may set off a disturbing chain reaction that could knock the entire organism, or relationship, or business organization, or project -- off balance. On the other hand, we can set off a benevolent, healing chain reaction if we deal with the problem correctly and carefully.

But how do we know the correct way of handling it? How do we know what the cause of the problem is?

One afternoon I got an incredibly excruciating headache -- a rare experience for me. When no meditation or accupressure helped, I just gave up and let go. I lay there on the sofa in desperation and shouted, "Okay, let me know whatever I need to know. What's my lesson for the day?"

Then, as fast as the pain had seized me, the pain left...and I gave birth to a realization: you do not necessarily have to know or define the problem for it to be solved. It can be resolved spontaneously through w h o l i s t i c   t r e a t m e n t .

Remember our discussion in Chapter 1 about the limitation of words? (If you don't , go back and read it.) Similarly, with a problem or a disease, we do not need to limit the healing with our conscious, ego-dominated insistence that we must diagnose the problem before it can be solved or healed. And we certainly do not want to restrict the improvement to what we only know. There may be problems or causes we do not consciously know about.

I used to wait until I had "all the facts" before I took decisive action, or before I allowed my plans to materialize. To my frustration, the more I learned, the more I researched, the more I tried to satisfy my insecure mind with "sure" answers and guarantees, the more I found I did not know and the more I learned to take nothing for granted.

A "lazy" parapsychological formula

Since we do not consciously perceive and know everything, let us give up the addiction that we must know everything. Let us recognize and humbly accept the limitation of our human minds. Having done that, we shall be able to free ourselves and open up to the realization of the unlimitedness of our human souls.

Through our soul, which is linked with the Universal Consciousness, we can know everything. But this knowledge may be, in large, unconscious. Yet, it can benefit us if we allow it to flow through us spontaneously and naturally.

As we evolve and expand our awareness, we will become more conscious of this "hidden knowledge." We may -- we can -- use it right now for healing, for problem solving; for goal realization of any kind.

WE CAN HEAL EVEN IF WE DO NOT KNOW WHAT IS WRONG AND WHAT TO DO ABOUT IT!   We are so accustomed to "sound" research, "certain" diagnosis and "responsible" treatment, that it may seem reckless and frightening to us to simply flow with the movement of Cosmic Intelligence as expressed through our inner guidance within our individual centers.

I do not suggest that we dismiss research and science as useless. It certainly can be used as a potent tool of cumulative conscious data that can be communicated and taught and kept alive and growing. The cosmic inspiration received by geniuses such as Einstein, (the scientist) Brahms (the composer) and Da Vinci (the artist-inventor) should not be dismissed or suppressed, either.

The marvelous, omnipotent Cosmic Intelligence is available to all of us whether we receive it via our dreams -- consciously or not -- through instinctive body cell consciousness, through "sudden" inspiration or through meditation.   CONSCIOUSLY OR UNCONSCIOUSLY, WE CHANNEL IT TO BUILD OR DESTROY, OR TO KILL.

Therefore, in order to heal the easy, "lazy" way, direct this energy Wholistically with the will, the belief and the request that it will flow to whatever area or dimension of the organism or its environment past, present and future that needs harmonizing and revitalizing.

Environmental Psychicommunications
How to get abundant healing from many directions

Everything in this beautiful cosmos of ours can be used as a symbol and transceiver of healing love-light.   Feel the loving, healing warmth of the sun.   Let yourself go in the calming blue of the skies. Ride on the elevating clouds.   Breathe in the power of the winds.   Let the mighty sea shape your body.   Recharge your being with the heat rising from the sand.   Behold the robust beauty of the trees.   Smell the purifying tenderness of the flowers.   Fill yourself with the youthful waters of life....

We can go on and on. ....   We can receive healing and guidance through nature, and we can send it...to our loved ones, to people, animals, plants, objects and projects we care about...and to the entire world through all of its kingdoms.

Even though using nature to send and receive healing love-light is perhaps the most romantic and harmonious way, we may also effectively use less beautiful means. We can transceive healing energies through the roar of airplanes, cars, and appliances; through sirens and explosions; through radio and TV, even through the move-ment of car wheels and the stench of smog.

You see, we can transform all sorts of energies -- expressed or carried through light, sound, smell or motion to work for us. We can use food, drink, emotions, touch, heat, cold, music, mass gatherings, exercise and love making, to focus powerful healing energies on ailments or conditions. Everything is energy and can be powerfully directed and focused if we develop our mental powers and "rewire" ourselves to safely handle such energies.

The means and examples are too many for the scope of this book. Even in my Wholistic 40-hour Self Improvement Training, we practice in depth only some means of Environmental Psychicommunications.

Here is one example of how Environmental Psychicommunications has worked for me: A few days after the New Year it was pouring rain, a condition uncommon in sun-spoiled Los Angeles. Los Ange-linos are either made out of sugar or else they are not accustomed to driving in the rain. It was quite likely that not a single soul would come to my Wednesday night Parapsychological Rap Session for Goal Realization and Problem Solving. I also had done nothing to promote the session that time because of my total involvement with the writing of this book. A few hours before 7:30 pm -- the starting time of my mini workshop -- I decided I didn't feel like sitting alone in my huge living room, before the fireplace, rapping with myself.

I took a few minutes to sit in quiet meditation among my beautiful plants and in front of the large painting of the Love Energy Transceiver of Self-Improvement which I had painted in a semi-trance state. As I asserted my oneness with the oval Love Energy Transceiver, my plants, and the entire universe, I could clearly hear the rain pouring outside and could practically see it and feel it with my expanded awareness through the walls and curtains of my living room.

I then generated love energy from my center (linked with the Infinite), and through the highly conductive rain drops and clouds, to all who needed some warmth and enlightenment that evening. I visualized the rain pouring my healing love upon all that could benefit from it, all who were in some way hurting and needed some extra good energy to cope with life and continue to evolve. And I asked that if some of the recipients of my radiated love-light needed some more direct energy, that they would find the courage to brave the cold, wet night and arrive here on time for a good session.

I was used to having from three to nine people for my Wednesday night sessions, on clear nights. Some people would always arrive late, and some would argue about my "right" as a spiritual teacher to charge "so much money" for the evening, namely $3.00!

Amazingly, on that dreary night, 30 people appeared -- some soaking wet -- all on time! Nobody greedily grouched about the $3.00. No one left the room before the session was over, not even to go to the bathroom. We had a marvelous, exciting discussion, especially when some people who were normally closed, opened up, released, and then brought out the hidden beauty within them. Everybody fully participated in the Wholistic meditation for goal realization and the problem solving with which we usually end the evening.

The evening turned out to be the most successful I can remember. Some people reported instantaneous healings! I, myself, got some additional insights and inspirations for my book; and felt as refreshed as though I had had a full night's sleep. There were additional reasons for the record success of the evening, but the "coincidence" of my pouring love through the rain and thunder should be open-mindedly considered.

This example could just as well be used in the next chapter dealing with healing of conditions. I used it here, first, to demonstrate further the connection between any condition, physical or financial, and how the basic Wholistic Healing principles encompass all conditions of disease, in all areas of life.

Applying the principle of Environmental Psychicommunications is especially useful when working on an "impossible" case. One of my local clients decided to give a life-saving gift to her sister in Alaska. She flew her to Los Angeles for 10 sessions with me.

The sister had much of her throat removed because of cancer. The cancer appeared to have been arrested, but the medical treatment left her vocal cords permanently damaged. The surgery left two gaping holes in her throat. One small hole was necessary for proper breathing and feeding (she was dependent on plastic tubes for liquid intake); the cther one, the larger one, was supposed to close after surgery, but did not.

Various surgeons tried grafting skin from other parts of the body in order to close the hole in her neck, but to no avail. As a last resort the sister was brought to me.

Of course, I guaranteed nothing, but said that with some help from above and with complete openness and trust on the part of the two sisters, everything -- however impossible it might appear -- was possible.

The first few sessions were spent on psychic diagnosis of the case and its causes: on Wholistic and emotional clearance. My initial hunch was immediately confirmed. The Alaskan sister had been very bitter. Before the cancer struck, she had misused her vocal cords to abuse her husband and others around her. Through relaxation, meditation and inducement of the flow of multi-color healing energies -- the sister opened up! She cleansed herself through "confession" and acceptance of responsibility. I considered that achievement as most important for her healing.

First, we worked together on the lessons that her cancer gave her, such as patience, positive thinking, "clean" language, self-image, and some karmic liberation. Subsequently, we focused and spread energies to get help from whatever direction was best for her to achieve harmony with life. Then we visualized the hole in her neck naturally closing in due time. Even when she wasn't there, I continued with this visualization in my daily meditations. This is called absent healing. Three days later, her sister called me from Palm Springs to tell me about a "miracle": the two sisters just "happened" to "bump into" a healer who proceeded to do some healing on the Alaskan sister. Next morning the sisters noticed that three quarters of the hole in the neck had closed!

Healing through the minds of the doctors on the case

In Wholistic Healing no stone is left unturned. The physicians and staff attending the case are, of course, crucial to the healing of the patient. Any thoughts crossing their minds, expressed or unexpressed, affects the balance of energies working through the patient. If a doctor believes that the case is lost, for example, this can contagiously contaminate not only the minds of the medical assistants and nurses, but also the mind of the patient -- even if the patient is in a coma.

Fortunately, contagious thought and belief flowing around the patient can also be optimistic and thus healing. Special attention, therefore, should be devoted to directing positive healing energies toward everyone connected with the case. Consequently, in our prayers and meditations, we should also ask that all doctors and staff (including those working at the information desk) will never lose hope. They should be enthusiastic about the chances of complete and speedy recovery of the patient no matter what the prognosis. They should mutually and increasingly reinforce their creative positiveness and radiate it to the patient and to each other in their thoughts, words, and actions. They should relentlessly be inspired on all levels and in all dimensions while working on the case -- whether they are around the patient or away -- while working, driving, sleeping, eating, drinking, eliminating, studying, praying or relaxing. There must be total focus on doing the right thing for the patient, with good for all concerned.

Doing that faithfully, a powerful magnetic field may be created around the case which could attract new discoveries and methods of treatment to allow Nature to heal the patient.

THOUGHT POLLUTION and how to reverse it -- Overcoming

negative attitude and resistance of a sick person and people around him

Thought pollution is worse, in my opinion, than air pollution. It can contaminate unaware minds with hate, bigotry, racism, fear, sorrow, and disease.

Thought pollution is not limited to established means of destructive propaganda. It can psychically poison minds and bodies. A mother can contaminate her infant with guilt; a father can poison his son with violence; whole families, gangs, organizations, nations can fall victim to a runaway psychic epidemic which is transmitted and reinforced through thought pollution.

Just as a Hitler can contaminate an entire nation, light can spread, too. It is the direction and balance of the play of energies; it is the Resultant of the Vectors of velocities, mass, and focus that determine whether we spread love or hate -- wholeness or destruction.

Because all energies come into play, every thought and every action count. Don't dismiss your contribution to the whole ocean of life as insignificant. It took a straw to break the camel's back. It may take just one prayer or meditation, or one benevolent thought to tip the balance in favor of recovery and harmony.

Each one of us can create accelerating and intensifying creative energies by transmitting good energies to people near us, then seeing the energies flow contagiously to many others, through the sick person, and then back to us -- greatly multiplied!

We, thus, snowball the healing energies until they overcome all resistance.

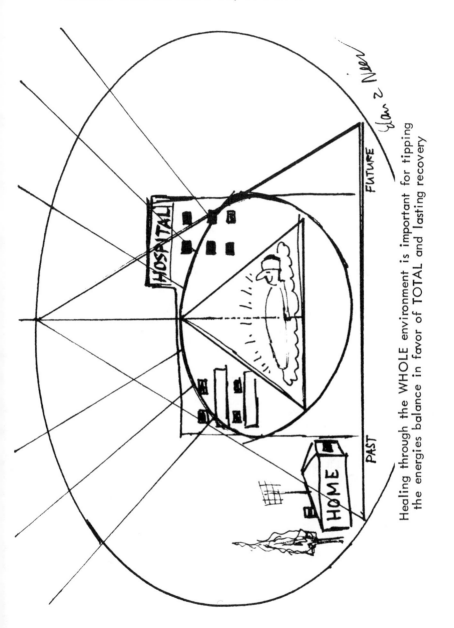

Healing through the WHOLE environment is important for tipping
the energies balance in favor of TOTAL and lasting recovery

After I completed training as a volunteer for Threshold Research Center on Death and Dying, I learned to never deny a sick person's feelings of anger or pain. Some of these people who were "doomed" to death were, indeed, bitter against their families and life in general. Yet, by listening to their complaints without preachingly telling them, for example, "Oh, you know things are not so bad. Your daughter really loves you. And the world being so full of flowers and sunshine, you truly don't have the right to hate it. And if you just let go, your pain will ease. It's mostly in your mind --" I drew their negativity out and away. They felt released and more peaceful. Then I would proceed to share my positiveness about life and death with them.

Basically, this technique of allowing the patient to express anger and pain is within the Cosmic Aikido approach as discussed in Chapter 2. Release makes room. This room can then be filled with positive, healing thoughts, conveyed through direct, or indirect communications: personal examples of positiveness and subliminal thought and feeling transference.

This subliminal "telecasting" can be made by hypnotic suggestion at the patient's bedside even while he is dozing or sedated. While he is awake, the positive suggestions should be made silently: mind to mind through auras, and through touch -- unless the patient has already released much of his anger and resistance and is, therefore, open to more direct communications.

If you feel that you absolutely have no power of communication with a stubborn, sick person wrapped in his self-destructiveness and agony, let me tell you something: YOU CAN COMMUNICATE HEALING LOVE ENERGIES EVEN TO SOMEONE WHO DOES NOT UNDERSTAND YOUR LANGUAGE, EVEN TO A SUICIDAL OLD DOG! I know it. I did it.

How to heal an old "dead" dog

In October, 1976 I was helping a Parkinson's disease victim. During the second session, the man who had not been able to walk, even with crutches, for two years, walked the width of my huge living room unaided. I was elated. I then recommended that the entire family should take my training so they could reinforce the healing process and reverse the destructive energies of illness that seemed to contaminate the whole family, as brother after brother was dying.

Most of the family was not receptive to spiritual healing and did not want to go through the sacrifice of time and money necessary to get full benefit from my Wholistic Self-Improvement and Oneness Intensive. So the idea was dropped.

Shortly thereafter, my client again stopped walking. I was so involved in wanting to help him permanently that I let some self-doubts creep into my mind.

To counteract this contamination from the destructive trend of events, I went to my favorite place of relaxation, meditation, and creation: the ocean. I was meditating while jogging on Venice Beach in California, when I was drawn to a small gathering. People were standing around a large, old, white dog. The dog was lying in the sand on its right side, its nose in the sand. No movement of sand was apparent around its nostrils.

I was told that the dog just suddenly collapsed and fell dead. I told the people I happened to be a psychic healer and that while I "specialized" in people, I once saved a small dog who was electrocuted, with mouth-to-mouth rescusitation.

The broad-minded Venitians told me I was welcome to work on the dead dog. Besides, the dog was not theirs.

Having nothing to lose but my dignity, I kneeled beside the body and placed my left hand on its left ribs and my right hand on its scalp. No motion or sound came from the dog. I closed my eyes and deeply inhaled healing energies from the Cosmos and sent them through my right hand into the dog, while drawing out negativities with my left. I felt the energies tingling through my body and through my hands. I started "hearing" a very slow, faint heart beat with my left hand.

Five minutes elapsed. The dog still showed no sign of breathing or moving. The heart beat was not improving at all.

I could feel the chilling stares of doubt from the small crowd around me. My own ego was acting up again, as a cold sweat of embarrassment and self-consciousness was budding on my forehead. I wished I were a Master, oblivious to what others thought of me. I wished they would go away!

In a few seconds the small crowd dispersed. Down there on the cool beach in winter remained a man and a dog and some curious seagulls. The dog's heart beat was slowing to almost nothingness and the roar of the great Pacific Ocean seemed to grow ominously. The breeze grew colder, too, and I smelled death.

I was fighting an urge to run away, to admit failure, to listen to Mommie who admonished me I was "in the wrong business."

But another part of me, my Higher Self, was grabbing me by the knees with the cool, moist sand and warning me not to permit my ego and false self take control.

I knew there was no time to lose. I talked to the dog in English and in the Holy Language, Hebrew. But the dog would not respond. I told it I loved it and wanted to play with it. Dead silence!

And then, it hit me: the realization that the dog had no will to live, nothing to live for.

With a desperate Biblical passion, I turned my closed eyes to Heaven with the plea: "If you want me to continue with my New Age mission, and if you also want me to continue to help people heal, show me -- right now -- that I can help this dog. Otherwise, I shall quit!!"

I knew I was playing with fire. I knew I was a small human being challenging the mighty mission. But something within me urged me to live dangerously. If my ancestor Israel could survive it, so could I. I felt the juices stirring within me. I felt waves of passion melting energy blocks within my human vehicle and releasing cumulative rage.

A thought flashed in my mind, curling my back with an electric charge and straightening it up again: "If you were a dog, what would motivate you to want to live?" "Another dog of the opposite sex," came the answer as quick as a flash.

I looked down at the dog. Ascertaining it was a male, I knew I had to arouse a desire for a bitch in its mind. But how? I couldn't lose time trying to explain my thoughts to it in English or Hebrew. And I didn't think French would help either. I needed to immediately transfer the excitement of life and its perpetual expression through sex to the dog, or it would die momentarily.

"The shortest communication between two minds is direct communication," flashed the instruction through my mind. I took a deep breath from the Cosmos and projected my mind into the dog's. I wondered what kind of a female dog it fancied. To play it safe, I visualized three bitches: one tall, long-haired, blond; one medium and white, and one small and black -- with curly hair. I felt my dog-awareness getting excited with expectation of fun and games.... The whole process took a few seconds, like in a dream. I felt my hands being pushed. I opened my eyes and there stood my canine

patient. Without stopping to thank me with a dripping lick, or at
least wiggle its tail goodbye, the dog was off running. I followed
its direction and lo, and behold: at a distance along the shore, I
saw three dogs of varied sizes!

I closed my eyes again. The cold breeze mixed my tears of
joy and thanksgiving with the chilly vapor of the crashing waves.
But cold I was not. A warm tingling throughout my body was
telling me that my tears were reuniting with the ocean...homecoming.
I knew a cycle in my life had just closed and a new one had begun.
I knew that my prayer to serve humanity was being accepted through
the Seven Kingdoms of the Universe.

Spontaneous remission and how to make it stick

My "mission" as a psychic healer started when I met a
government auditor during a course I took under Ken Key of the
Living Love Center. The auditor was eager to take my "infant"
Wholistic 40-hour Self-Improvement Workshop based on some comments
I made about harmony with life. He wanted to help his ex-girl
friend who was dying in St. Vincent's Hospital with a glioma seated
deep within her brain. The cancerous tumor was so large that it could
not be totally removed. She was given about seven days to live.

Since there was not much time to lose, the auditor (who was
quite psychic and an evolved soul) asked me to save his friend's life.
I told him I was a New Age teacher but not a healer. He insisted I
was both. Reluctantly, I agreed to try to heal his dying friend if he
secured permission.

When I entered her room, Death greeted me as if it owned the
place. The young woman's face was white. I was told she could not
talk anymore or open her eyes, and that she was being fed intra-
venously. I sat beside her bed staring at a skeletal head. According
to a photograph I was shown, she had once been quite attractive.
Somehow I felt that she was encouraging Death.

As I intently stared at her, wondering how to reach her
cancerous brain, she opened one of her eyes, which her friend
considered a miracle. I felt a life force flowing into and through
me and into her eye, like an aggressive missionary placing his foot
in the door in order to prevent it from being closed in his face. I
grabbed her left hand, which was as cold as if it belonged to a
corpse, and let her draw through it all the love she seemed to crave
...as if she had been starving for love all of her 32 years. The
hand began getting warmer and warmer, and the other eye opened.

I wasn't sure she could hear me through her ears, or understand me consciously through her deteriorating mind, but I talked anyway.   I talked with a soothing but firm voice; I talked with my imagination, transmitting pictures into her mind; I talked with my hands and aura, caressing and permeating her dwindling being with love and hope.   I talked about her accepting and releasing her angry oppressive parents.   I talked about her right and desire to choose her own path in life.   I talked about her fulfillment and about the ecstacy of life awaiting outside, if she just learned from her bitter lessons to think freely and guiltlessly.

Three days later I visited her once more.   This was my last visit.   Her parents were waiting outside the room as I entered.   She was well enough to hug me and to demonstrate her hearty appetite by eating the whole hospital lunch.   She talked, too, and told me about her dreams.   As I was helping her interpret her dreams, I was guided to lead her through a healing meditation.   We used her dreams to create new dreams about the book she was going to write, about the piano lessons she was going to take.   She was relaxing, with a pretty smile on her flushed face.

Death seemed to have been banished.   Yet, when the woman's father, like an immature child, jealously demanded his daughter's love and attention, I chillingly realized that Death was still on call.

Only a few days later she was discharged from the hospital.   In a meditative group healing from a distance, my Wholistic Self-Improvement class, which involved the ecstatic, smiling auditor who talked me into my "first healing," was thoroughly washing her brain, scrubbing the tumor off, and bathing the brain with a healing love-light.   In subsequent psychic "diagnoses," my budding psychic students and graduates could no longer find any tumor.   The patient appeared to have what Dr. Thelma Moss of the University of California would call a spontaneous remission.

Months passed, and the young woman resumed a "normal" life. She walked, ate, read, spoke coherently, wrote...and was kept a prisoner by her parents!   They would not let her friend, the auditor, (who was by now one of my prize graduates) visit her or take her out because of his "evil occult ways;" and whenever I tried to cheer her up over the phone, they would hang up on me.   Her physician expressed broadmindedness in his letter to me.   He wrote: "What is impressive is there was a distinct change in the patient's attitude in her 'will to live'...and "a significant change in her attitude towards her illness, towards the people around her, and towards herself."   But even this advanced and courageous doctor allowed contamination of the healing process with the thought expressed in his letter: "On a probability basis I would think improvement was temporary, but I certainly was impressed...."

About seven months later, I became restless thinking of this young woman. I inquired about her from my graduate auditor who said he was still not allowed to communicate with her, except, of course, psychically, but he assured me she was completely back to normal according to a mutual girl friend. I called her home and pleaded with her mother to let me speak to my "patient," but the mother shouted that her daughter was alright, warning me never to call again. I called the physician's office and had a lengthy conversation with his partner, who said that she never really believed the whole thing, and that whatever improvement occurred in the patient was due to the medical treatment and some lucky coincidences. She went on to say that it was unheard of that a patient with such a huge tumor on the brain would recover, and that it was just a matter of time before the patient would certainly expire. In tears I pleaded with her to ask her partner, who was obviously more romantic and open, to call me as soon as he returned to the office.

Shortly after, he called. He was receptive and sympathetic. He promised he would ask the parents to allow me to visit his patient. Keeping his word, he reported back to me that the parents adamantly refused to allow their daughter any communication either with me or my graduate. He expressed a good understanding of the psychological problems between the parents and the daughter which had provoked her attempt at mental suicide which took the form of a brain cancer, since she wasn't strong enough to "free" herself constructively. Because the parents were not abusing their daughter physically, there was nothing else he could legally do, except make his recommendations.

A few weeks later she made good her escape. According to her girl friend, one evening after a "normal fight" with her parents she told them, "I am going away and I am going to come back, but not to you. I am going to come back to the flowers...as a beautiful butterfly." Next morning, she was dead.

TO MAKE HEALING LAST, WE NEED TO REMOVE THE CAUSE OF THE DISEASE. If we simply cut a weed, it will grow back to constrict the growth of flowers. If we kill it with chemicals, other plants, animals, or even ourselves may be poisoned. We may pull out the weed by the roots. This may be useful, if in the process we don't pull or damage other plants. However, if we could remove soil and environmental conditions conducive to the growth of the weed and provide harmonious conditions for the growth of the intended useful plants, we would have the ideal conditions.

In Wholistic Healing, we don't just "heal." We maintain harmonious conditions so that the disease will have no reason to return. This is why each one of us believing in the "miracles" of Wholistic Healing should enlighten all those who come in touch with us. As the cliche says, "the life you save may be your own!"

Protecting yourself while healing others

I often meet psychic healers who complain of being drained by their patients. I also know of cases where students of various mind expansion courses developed the very problems they wanted to heal.

In one case, for example, a lady who took one of the commercially most successful courses in mind probing, was trying to psychically "see" another woman of her age who had a breast removed. Because she had difficulties visualizing, the instructor's wife told her to project herself, instead, as if on a mirror. Doing so, without being properly cleared, centered, and free of her intellectual and mental blocks -- the student inadvertently programmed cancer upon herself: within six months she lost her breast without being able to help the person she was supposed to help.

This is why, at Self-Improvement Institute, we emphasize cleansing of the mind, soul and body; centering; releasing; and developing harmony and rhythm with life -- instead of stressing the importance or superiority of technique. When we clear, when we are "rewired" for New Age energies, any technique works better. And there is no one technique which is best for everyone all the time with every situation.

So, the first precaution in healing others is CLEANSE, PURIFY AND CENTER YOURSELF BEFORE YOU ATTEMPT ANY HEALING. The cleansing will remove the toxins or negativities within your mind which may attract negativities from the patient. It will also allow both the healing energies you send and the negative energies you draw from the client and out of you, to flow through you unhindered. The centering will allow you to ground out of your system intense healing forces that may short-circuit your system and/or negative energies you need to get out of the patient and out of your body. The centering will also assure that all healing love energies flow through you -- through your entire center -- thereby filling you with health and blessing before they go to your client.

Don't worry about being "selfish." If you follow the Biblical rule of "Love thy neighbor as thyself," you will have no trouble: you start with yourself. You fill yourself with love energy through your own center, which is linked with the Cosmos. You establish an abundant inner flow of love energy. Only then are you ready to share it with your patient.

When you establish such centered flow of energies, you program yourself to never give more healing life energies than you receive. YOU FILL YOURSELF WITH HEALING LOVE-LIGHT FIRST, AND THEN, AND ONLY THEN, YOU RADIATE THROUGH YOU THE ENERGY AS YOU HEAL OR ENHANCE YOURSELF IN THE PROCESS.

When you are filled with healing love-light, you tend to attract such energy from others. When you deal that way with a person in need, you induce that person's center to attract and generate healing love-light that will be healing him, as well as blessing you and others around.

This is the reason why, when I induce a healing or when I teach or lecture, I find myself increasingly more energetic and well. I accelerate the Great Life Force that flows through my central nervous system, and through my chakras (psychic centers) throughout my being, so that inevitably I, too, benefit from it as I effectively help others.

I have found the following practices to be good protection: meditate or pray before the healing. Surround yourself with protective light such as the Sii pyramid of light described at the end of Chapter 1. Program that you get 10-fold return in good health from the abundant universe for every bit of energy you expend. Light a candle for guidance and purification of the vibration. Place a glass of water nearby for further absorption of impurities. Shake your hands after meditation to clear out negative vibration. Avoid healing when you are fatigued or irritated. Build up your Self-Improvement Psychic Antibody.

The ultimate protection: Psychic Antibody

I stumbled upon this concept when I began to expand the phenomenon of the natural immunization the body builds.

You well know that a baby who grew in a sterile environment is much more vulnerable to "catching" all sorts of disease once suddenly exposed to the street, than the baby who grew in a dirtier environment. The second baby is immune. He took in enough germs to make his body familiar with the various diseases lurking in the street so that it built antibodies from within to balance and fight off disease.

I believe this antibody concept works on all levels of existence. Just as we can improve our immunity from typhus fever, by getting an injection of some typhus germs in our blood, we can immunize ourselves from accidents, negative energies, and all kinds of mishaps, including disease, by developing an awareness and acceptance of their existence.

Nietzsche once said, "A tree whose branches reach up to heaven should have roots reaching down to hell." This is the balance between the polarities that an independent, whole system can reach. If, instead of pretending that disease and evil do not exist, we accept life as is -- we can create a balance that will assure that nothing will catch us off guard; nothing will shock us. We then have such an expanded KNOWINGNESS, such a good intelligence-gathering system, that we are well prepared for every eventuality.   This protective awareness I call PSYCHIC ANTI-BODY, or you may call it Expanded Antibody, if you are prejudiced against the adjective psychic (if you are, study well Chapter 1).

Water and food healing and protecting

Everything we take into our systems, be it light, air, food, or water, can be used to heal us or protect us.

Take water. for example.   It is a potent conductor of electricity and sound.   It is magnetic to the extent that it attracts impurities and thus cleanses.   It can even draw smoke from a smoke-filled room if put in an open bowl.

If we accept and expand these natural characteristics of water, we can energize water even further: putting the glass of water in the sun, on a pyramid energizer; focusing on it with our minds, holding it in our hands -- any or all of the above.

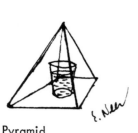

Pyramid

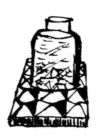

Pyramid Energizer

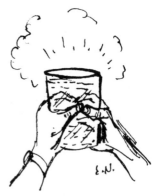

As we look into the water and touch the glass with both hands, we can meditate that the water will wash away the causes of the inharmonious condition, then magnetize the resulution of the problem and the toal healing. As we drink the water, we fill ourselves with the belief that the water will circulate the message of cleansing and blessing through our brains and bodies, attracting divine order and healing.

Our systems consist mainly of water, so why not bless the water we drink or give?! And why not release impurities through it of mind, soul and body? (See earlier section on release.)

When I was on KFI radio station in October, 1976, answering questions about Wholistic Health, I demonstrated a simple water healing technique. Following is a typical testimonial letter I received after the program: "On Radio KFI one night Dr. Neev was helping an inquirer with some problem and he advised her to take a glass of water and project healing consciousness into the water, clasping it with both hands, touching each other and thinking as she drank, it was healing water of life.... I did so, as I had a bad case of indigestion, and it was healed instantly."   Flora Lind

While I was projecting healing energies into the water for all who drank it to heal, I knew that through the phenomenon of oneness discussed in Chapter 7, I was effectively healing all water regardless of barriers of space. You can also transcend barriers of time by programming (or treating) that wherever the person whom you want to help drinks water (or any drink for that matter), the water will be energized with the healing powers you projected into it.

You can also put a glass of water near your bed charging the water to cleanse your being and environment from all negativities during sleep or sickness. Then pour it ceremoniously into the toilet once a day.

Water healing lends itself beautifully to animal and plant healing as well. It also works in conjunction with color healing.

Any creative or benevolent thought that you inject into anything you take in can help. You can now see how prayers and blessings over food and water, and the advice that eating should be done in a pleasant and relaxed atmosphere, make so much more sense!

Color healing

In Self-Improvement Institute we include the seven rays of the rainbow in our Wholistic approach. You see, each color has a different energy frequency which affects one aspect or another of your personality and works through certain chakras along your spine and head.

Ray 1 is red and controls the chakra (psychic center) at the base of the spine. It is the color of vitality and is also helpful in treating anemia, paralysis and circulation.

Ray 2 is orange and controls the chakra in the spleen. It is the color of coordinating and freeing vital energies and is also helpful for treating the spleen, kidneys and psychosomatic paralysis.

Ray 3 is yellow and controls the solar plexus -- the "brain center" of the nervous system. It is the color of bright mental activity and is also useful for treating skin, nerves and circulation.

Ray 4 is green and controls the cardiac chakra. It is the color of balance, harmony and abundance, and is also useful for treating cancer, heart, headaches and flu.

Ray 5 is blue and controls the throat chakra. It is the color of calming spirituality and is helpful for treating the throat, children's sicknesses, insomnia, and shock.

Ray 6 is indigo and controls the third eye chakra (at the pineal gland). It is the color of purification and higher consciousness and understanding, and is useful for the treatment of ears, nose, eyes and throat.

Ray 7 is violet and controls the crown chakra at the top of the head. It is the color of inspiration and idealism and is helpful in treating the mind, rheumatism, meningitis, kidney and bladder.

We can use the color rays individually or in combination to heal various conditions through charging water in colored glass and/or or our imagination ; through colored lamp radiation or colored windows; through food and drink of various colors; through inhaling or absorbing colors in our imagination; through breathing color on the area or person to be healed; and through wearing colored clothes.

The simplest Wholistic way is to ask in meditation, and know that the Super Consciousness will radiate the necessary colors in the proper intensity, length of time, and blend, according to the individual need at the time -- for maximal and fastest restoration of wholeness -- with good to all concerned now and in the long run.

When we are in the Sii pyramid of white light, we just know that our Higher Self blends and focuses the seven rays exactly according to our needs.

Other forms of healing, and some legal warning

There are many other forms of healing not directly discussed here, such as healing by touch (healing hands, accupressure, etc.), through special spiritual dieting (such as through herbs, sprouting and raw food eating), via fasting, by faith (such as in the name of Christ, in spiritual churches), through white magic, and through yoga and other exercises.

Some forms of healing may be superior to others in some cases. The thing to consider, however, is that there may be no one way which is best for everyone, all of the time, with every problem. This is why Wholistic Healing is the safest and most comprehensive approach. It allows for any specific form of healing -- from the conventional medical treatment to primitive voodoo -- to work better and in harmony with other treatments.

But whatever you choose for yourself -- or for others, if you are a healer -- be cautious not to take anything for granted; not to conflict with, or disrupt, medical treatment; and not to practice against the law of your government.

WHOLISTIC HEALING REQUIRES WHOLESOME AND HARMONIOUS PERFORMANCE WITH ALL -- AND THIS CERTAINLY INCLUDES YOUR PHYSICIAN AND THE LAW.

CHAPTER 5

HEALING CONDITIONS, FINANCES, RELATIONS...
EVEN THE WORLD!

How important and influential are you really?

As we move on with this book, we may realize that it is guided
Wholistically: cycles are closing, enough pieces are being put into
place to create a whole new picture, and the understanding and use of
concepts are being expanded and contracted through cyclic repetition to
encompass more and more and more....

In Chapter 4 we discussed how the last straw can break the camel's back through environmental interplay of cumulative energies. YOU ARE IMPORTANT. YOU ARE INFLUENTIAL. YOU CAN DESTROY OR START DESTRUCTION. OR YOU CAN BUILD OR START BUILDING.

Naturally, the first one to suffer or to benefit as you direct the destructive or creative energies is you.

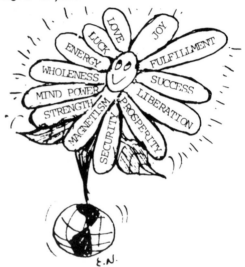

Who is responsible and how to profit from ENLIGHTENED SELFISHNESS

As a prerequisite to Wholistic Healing we must stop blaming others for our condition or expecting others to bail us out of trouble. As Rabbi (meaning teacher in Hebrew) Hillel said in Pirke Avot (the Hebrew Sayings of the Sages) about 2,000 years ago: "If I am not for myself, who will be? And being for my own self (only) what am I? And if not now, when?"

These profound words encompass all of Wholistic Healing: I take responsibility for myself, because through my center (mind, central nervous system and power centers or psychic centers or chakras), I am directing the Life Force for good or for bad. When blessing comes my way, I attract it through my link with the cosmos. If a curse comes, I attract it, too, consciously or unconsciously. When I attract both, it is because I am not whole enough yet, and the conflicting selves within me are attracting what they need or deserve according to their states of consciousness.

But since we are part of a whole and cannot escape this reality, let us realize that if we think of ourselves only, we are unnaturally trying to cut ourselves off from the abundant whole and its great benefits. (See sub-chapters on Environmental Psychicommunications, and on Protecting yourself, in Chapter 4, plus the entire discussion of the law of Oneness in Chapter 7.)

If you read me carefully, you know by now that I am strongly against the type of unbalanced altruism where you put others before yourself. However, I am certainly for ENLIGHTENED SELFISHNESS or EXPANDED CENTEREDNESS.

If you couple this Enlightened Selfishness with a good sense of timing and also comprehend Hillel's rhythmic concept of "if not now, when?" you are in possession of a powerful prescription for harmony with life and total success and fulfillment!

Giving and receiving ... the wonders of energy exchange

If we apply Hillel's prescription to everyday life, we soon realize that it facilitates a smoother and more abundant flow of energy through us. We give more freely of ourselves and we receive more freely. Translated into more specific benefits, we become more energetic, enthusiastic, lovable, better communicators and learners, and more healthy, resourceful and rich! Spiritually speaking, we accelerate our evolution, fan our inspiration, multiply our healing powers and unite with the Source! Can we ask for more?!

The incredible power of expanding your goal to include others

If you apply to your planning the triple wisdom prescription of the Hebrew sage Hillel, you'll find an unfailing tool for success, spiritually, socially and financially.

Take any personal goal you have right now. Let's work on it for faster and more complete realization. Ask yourself, how can other people benefit from the success of my goal? What's in it for others?

If you discover some benefits for others (others could be customers and employees or partners or the entire economy and society), expand on these benefits and fill your awareness with them.

If you do not find worthwhile benefits for others, expand your goal to include them, for your own good. BY INCLUDING OTHERS, YOU INTENSIFY THE ENERGIES PULLING AND PUSHING TOWARD THE REALIZATION OF YOUR GOAL.

Even if your goal includes the good of others, make sure the fact is paramount in your awareness and that in meditation you perceive all those "others" sharing in the joys of your success.

FOR MY OWN GOAL EXPANSION, I ENVISION THIS BOOK HELPING PEOPLE ALL OVER THE WORLD. This will bring me much spiritual and financial reward, which I wish to return in the form of creating the International Center of Communication for World Leaders and World Peace (ICCWLWP) at the United Nations and away. Leaders in conflict will be helped there to reconcile differences, and future diplomats will be accredited as expert peace makers. Thus I hope to help heal world consciousness for universal harmony.

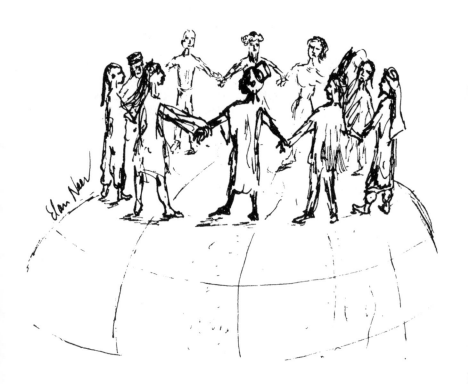

How to hook your energies onto mighty benevolent currents to speed up harmony, success, fulfillment and prosperity

Now that we are warming up with the understanding of the flow of energies, let us expand our understanding of it a bit further. Carefully observe others and their goals; search for a common denominator.

If you are a leader of any sort -- parent, teacher, manager, salesperson, politician, officer, and the like -- find the needs and goals of your people. See how you can help them realize their goals as you realize yours. Assist them to expand their goals to reinforce each other's success energies -- yours included. This is the secret of the most harmonious motivation.

Now go even further. Raise your consciousness and expand your awareness. Think of your community as a whole, consisting of your town, city, state, country -- the whole cosmos! Think of the past, present and future as one. Tune into the trends of cosmic evolution and join your energies with the highest and best.

You may maintain your uniqueness and personal integrity even if you join the New Age mighty currents of liberation and world peace. In fact, your own individual mission in life can be fulfilled faster if it is in harmony with New Age energies. Why dissipate energy, struggling along a dirt road because of some monomaniacal desire for privacy and individual grandeur if you can reach your destination by a more comfortable drive? Or take a jet and fly with the established, powerful energies part of the way, later taking an individual route. By then, you will be so much closer to your destination and full of energy and good will toward others.

Leaning, expectations, addictions, ego and fear -- the cripplers

Riding on the New Age currents may not be so easy for everyone as it may seem at first. There are strict passenger regulations: light baggage! You must travel light the path of life.

To travel light, we must drop off excess weight such as leaning on others, heavy expectation, "unbreakable" habits, irrational fears, and the tyranny of our restless, biased INTELLECTUAL MIND controlled by our ego.

Shedding these burdens will allow us to see beyond the petty goals in front of our noses. And it will richly reward us with an exhilarating sense of freedom to move and grow, freedom to think and create, freedom to enjoy ourselves and enjoy seeing others enjoy themselves!

How a salesman doubled his income in one month

One of the graduates of my Wholistic 40-hour Self-Improvement Workshop is an insurance broker. He took the course with his wife in order to learn to relax better in the face of mounting business pressures.

At the end of the training he wrote, "I feel as if a heavy burden has been lifted off my heart." A month and a half later he wrote, "Since taking the course I've been having a tremendous growth in my insurance business. For the month of June, the volume of business doubled over the previous month. For the month of July, the volume of business is higher than June." He later reported that business became a pleasure since he removed the anxiety out of it and was just pouring love into creating the best insurance plans to fit the needs of his clients, without worrying about his plans being rejected, his ego being hurt, or his time being lost. Consequently, he now gets more done in less time. His magnetism has grown to the point where clients now seek him.

Affirmations and Meditation for healing conditions

Bring yourself into a meditative state as in the end of Chapter 1. Affirm from within your center: "I tune myself to the highest vibrations of the universe. Through the light, I claim my share of the abundant universe. I pour love into my work and relations without anxiety about the outcome. I accept in advance whatever the results of my efforts, knowing I always learn from all experiences, including set-backs, and always move cheerfully forward without taking anything for granted. I replace all addictive expectations with a grand, unconditional expectancy of good in due time, with benefits to all concerned and in harmony with life.

I serve my clients, students, or employers with love and devotion -- for my own good. I expand my interests and goals to include all around me and throughout the world.

I ask for Divine Order and guidance so that I fulfill my mission in life in harmony with the missions of others and within the grander missions.

I want the world to be a better place for me to live in. I want to be in harmony with the rhythm and music of the Cosmos. To this end, I seek to enrich the world rather than deplete it -- to provide love and service to humanity in as modest or grand a way as I am guided to follow.

I ask to join the energies of the New Age to have a maximal use of all my talents to bring about immediate and lasting success, wealth, health and happiness to me, and through me to my family, friends, affiliates and the entire Universe. I am a universal person seeking to bring out the best in me and others for peace, prosperity, fulfillment and joy.

Visualize now a tremendous rainbow across the heavens coming out of the Love Energy Transceiver and surrounding the globe. Duplicate the rainbow-encircled globe in the center of your head.

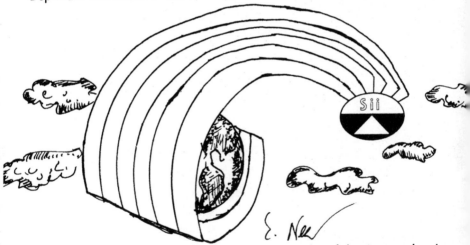

Let the rainbow wrap itself once around the globe in your head and continue down your spine all the way to your feet and the floor.

Know that you are one with the harmonious vibrations of the universe and that all good passes through you. And so it is.

WRITE HERE YOUR EXPANDED GOAL:

CHAPTER 6

FATE OR FREE WILL? AND SO WHAT?

An ancient Hebrew solution to an age-old argument

Some people are off balance in their bodies, emotions, relations or finances because of resisting and fighting life. They cynically reject anything beyond their comprehension. They believe the world owes them a living. They will not accept or respect the Universal Laws and thus abuse the environment and their own bodies and souls, as well as others. They live for themselves only and believe in no power above them.

At the other extreme are the fatalists who believe there is nothing they can do. Whatever will be will be. They run to astrologers and fortune tellers to predict their futures, and they limit their lives by the fear of the future and by their feelings of helplessness.

People on either extreme are vulnerable to disharmony in all areas of life. About 2,000 years ago Rabbi Akibah, the Hebrew Sage said in The Sacred Sayings of the Fathers, "Everything is foreseen, yet freedom of choice is given; and the world is judged by grace, yet everything is according to the amount of the work."

This saying, if properly understood, can resolve the whole conflict between fatalists and free willers: yes, everything is foreseen. There are Universal Laws that are unbreakable such as the laws of cause and effect and the law of polarity. Within the Universal Laws there is predictability.

BUT WITHIN THE PREDICTABLE LAWS OF NATURE, THERE IS MUCH ROOM TO VIBRATE, PULSATE AND GROW. THERE IS A FREE WILL. And it is your free choice whether you are poor or rich, ill or well, miserable or happy. With work on yourself, you can materialize your choice.

Balance

To be fulfilled we must maintain a balance between when we let go and when we interfere and apply our wills. We may miss a lot if we apathetically let life fly by, yet we may miss a lot if we unnecessarily enslave ourselves with burning desires.

How do we achieve this balance?

Passive and Active Harmony

When we let go and float on the currents of life unharmed, we experience PASSIVE HARMONY.

When we learn how to use the waves and the winds to go in the direction we will, we experience ACTIVE OR CREATIVE HARMONY.

In basic meditation you learn to passively relax, empty your mind, transcend the five senses, and allow the Great Life Force to flow through you. This can be very helpful for spontaneous healing of all conditions, for revitalization, and for spontaneous protection.

When I was a life guard during my early college days in Canada, I was also teaching swimming to beginners. I taught them how to float first. Having learned to float -- which is being in Passive Harmony -- I taught them how to swim.

Swimming well, with minimum fatigue -- especially in the ocean -- is being in Creative Harmony. If we are merely in Passive Harmony, the ocean of life may take us to beautiful places. But since with our powerful minds we can focus energies and become CREATORS, or at least CO-CREATORS, we achieve Creative Harmony as we add direction and purpose to our living.

True, with Creative Harmony we stand a greater chance of meeting opposition or making "mistakes" than with Passive Harmony. With Creative Harmony, more of our conscious awareness and WILL come into play. But as we learn from our "mistakes" and "failures", as we overcome opposition -- we grow faster. It is like developing muscles via isometric exercise.

The secrets of willing and letting

We are closing another cycle of comprehension. TO BE IN FULL HARMONY WITH LIFE, TO BE WHOLE IN BODY, MIND AND SOUL, WE MUST FUNCTION IN BOTH PASSIVE AND CREATIVE STATES OF HARMONY. We must learn when to passively let go and when to creatively will. I like to compare this concept with swimming the breast stroke, where by forcing our arms back, we propel ourselves forward. As we let go and float with the momentum, we regain strength for the next willed action.

CHAPTER 7

THE MASTER KEY--

THE UNIVERSAL LAW OF ONENESS

The amazing Yo-Yo of the Yang and the Yin

I continuously stress that we are subject to the relativity of all values. The ancient Chinese called this phenomenon the Yang and the Yin. (Also see Chapter 3, ..."Getting into the swing of life".)

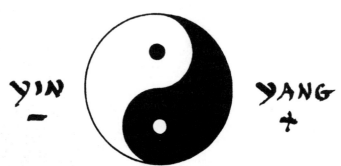

The YANG is the male tendency of CONTRACTION and the +
polarity in electrical current. The YIN is the female tendency of
EXPANSION and the – (minus) polarity in electricity. Although the
YANG and the YIN are in tension, they complement and counter-
balance each other. As the Kybalion (the teachings of Hermes)
states: "Everything is Dual; everything has poles; everything has its
pair of opposites; like and unlike are the same; opposites are
identical in nature, but different in degree; extremes meet; all truths
are but half-truths; all paradoxes may be reconciled."

THIS RECONCILIATION OF THE OPPOSITES IS THE MASTER
KEY OF CREATIVITY, HARMONY, WELLNESS, AND WHOLENESS.
IT IS THE SECRET OF ONENESS.

The reconciliation takes place as the YANG and the YIN
infiltrate each other's very center in an intercourse of life's
vibration and pulsation, causing an orgasmic realization that AT
CENTER ALL THINGS ARE ONE.

Practical aspects of Oneness -- You don't have to believe. They
work anyway!

The universe is one. It encompasses worlds within worlds
within worlds. Man is part of everything and everything is part of
man.   Man is an integral part of the universe and the universe is
within man.   Man contains the planets, stars, land, and sea. Our
wholeness depends on our conscious and unconscious acceptance of
this fact. Awareness of it will help us flow with life.

Our breath is like the wind. If we habitually try to constrict
it, it will not bring us the seeds of blessing we need or blow the
"smog" out of our systems.

Our blood flows like the rivers streaming toward the sea which, in turn, evaporates into clouds which, via rain, replenish the rivers.

Flowing with the cycle of life and loving the Creation with all our being makes our being whole.

A person who tries to deny his Oneness with all -- who violates Nature -- is thus attempting suicide. For example, if you turn with hate on a group of people, you are turning on yourself, because you are part of them. Hitler, therefore, was not simply destroyed by the "forces of good" -- he destroyed himself!

Similarly, even if less dramatically, we are not victim to disease, poverty, mishaps and suffering -- we bring them upon ourselves. IT IS OUR FREE CHOICE TO EXTRICATE OURSELVES FROM CRIPPLING CIRCUMSTANCES, EVEN IF WE WERE BORN INTO THEM! As long as we hold ourselves slaves to habits or "circumstance" as an easy alibi, we are in contempt of our Oneness with the abundant universe...and we suffer for that.

Have we left God out?

'Til now I haven't mentioned God by name. As discussed in Chapter 1, words can be limiting. Whatever your belief, what is, IS!

So if you are an agnostic or atheist, I don't want you to miss the fun of harmony. Maybe you believe in electric currents instead of in God. Maybe you just use different words to describe what other people call God or one aspect of God.

This is why in Sii we accept students of all faiths and function non-dogmatically. We believe in fostering New Age natural growth from within the individual's center according to his or her level of understanding and evolutionary growth.

Personally, I grew from agnosticism to believing in one omnipotent, all-encompassing God. I do, however, accept humbly and lovingly the fact that various individuals and groups perceive Providence according to their perspective, awareness, language and thinking processes.

I feel that optimum harmony is experiencing within, a oneness with God.

Using God to be well?!

I now understand what the Biblical affirmation of my ancestors "the Lord is One" really meant: it is the affirmation of the Oneness in the Universe.

The importance of this realization is so great for our Wholeness that the Bible commanded: "Thou shalt love the Lord, thy God with all thy heart, with all thy soul, and with all thy might." IF WE UNDERSTAND GOD AS ONE AND BEING EVERYWHERE IN AND AROUND US -- LOVING GOD IS THE GREATEST, MOST POTENT "FORMULA" OF WHOLISTIC HEALING.

If we worship God as some being in the sky outside of us, we may get some benevolent inspiration. But to be whole, we must love God everywhere with our entire being -- mind, soul, and body -- all of the time..."when thou sittest in thy house, when thou walkest by the way, when thou liest down, and when thou risest up."

Such powerful all-embracing affirmation of our Oneness is certain to channel such Godly love-light through our beings and environment that astonishing protection and healing can result as we get closer to the Source -- without even consciously knowing anything about healing or the causes of the ailment.

During one of my Wholistic Oneness Self-Improvment Workshops, we saw this love power in action:

After about 30 hours of intense cleansing and centering, I was guided to go through a most potent Kabalistic Mantra with my students. I knew the group could safely channel the Divine Healing Force and I very much wanted to help a young lady who, because of a stroke she had suffered 13 years ago, could not control her right hand or breathe through her nose. The class and I built up Love energy through Kabalistic means I then synthesized, using Eastern and Western techniques. The focus of the energies was our Unity With the Source -- Our Oneness.

After some vigorous group energizing where some students experienced emotional release, each student went "out" on an individual "journey" under my supervision (and our spiritual guides).

As I was waiting for my students, who were in deep meditation on the floor, to return to the "objective" world in the "here and now," I was praying silently to God for my students, especially for that lady who needed it most.

Suddenly I heard her voice squealing in the dark: "I don't believe it! I don't believe it!"

I turned the lights on and saw my student surrounded by her loving classmates on the floor, holding her healed hand for all to see.

"You do believe it!!" I thundered at the student who was drenched in tears of joy. "We do believe it!" echoed my students. And then my student realized she was also able to breathe again through her nose!

All of us who experienced the "miracle" of Oneness with God will never be cynical again. Amen.

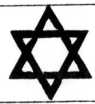

The triangle pointing up represents Man striving toward the Source. The one pointing down represents the Source reaching toward Man. Interlaced, they connote Oneness.

The incredible ESP technique of diagnosing and healing from a distance

I purposely waited with this sub-chapter until now. In Wholistic Healing, it is important to transcend the limitations of what we know consciously. We can heal even if we don't know.

Now that you are sufficiently acquainted with this freeing notion, we can safely describe an amazing psychic phenomenon that works through the principle of oneness.

BY FOCUSING OUR AWARENESS OF OUR ONENESS ON AN ILL STRANGER, WE CAN EXPERIENCE HIM -- HOWEVER FAR AWAY -- TO THE DEGREE THAT WE CAN DESCRIBE HIM WITH ASTONISHING ACCURACY, AND PROCEED TO HELP HIM HEAL FROM A DISTANCE!

When I mentioned this fact in a public lecture on the Short Path to Self-Improvement, a member of my audience -- a professor -- said: "You look like an honest and intelligent clean-cut man. How can you make such a statement without expecting to insult the intelligence of fair-minded people?"

"Professor," I said, "if I told you 50 years ago that I have a box at home which can show me two men hopping on the moon, in living color, would you have believed me? Now you know it is true. So, if a man-made electronic device can transmit images in color all the way from outer space, doesn't it stand to reason that the far more sophisticated bio-computer, namely, our human mind, can get in touch with this intelligence floating everywhere?"

The professor walked out to avoid witnessing the demonstration I was about to give. I then knew what Galileo must have felt centuries ago!

In my classes we actually learn how to do it, safely and with great spiritual and physical benefits.

I'll give you an actual illustration of how it works.

The brother of one of my graduates was in the hospital, critically ill. His heart stopped a few times and the doctors didn't give him more than the night to live.

I gathered a small group of my students and we all went into a meditative state of mind. Then we projected the ill boy on a mental screen as we temporarily became one with his awareness. Having his first name only, the students were able to see him in their minds and describe him with details that left no doubt in his sister's mind (my graduate) that, indeed, he was the boy on their mental screens.

Furthermore, we unanimously saw problems with his heart and circulation. I was then psychically guided to direct the group to cleanse his heart and his entire body from the toxins killing him and to visualize him well and happy.

We then proceeded to talk to him from inside his brain -- as we were united with him in our oneness -- about his will to live and purpose in life. Then, we "treated" his doctors to be divinely guided and his family to be free from the emotional problems plaguing it.

Whether we did it or not, the next morning he was removed from the critical list and three days later was released from the hospital! And the entire family was going through deliberate soul searching and problem solving.

The ESP projection through oneness works equally well in describing dead people, which further proves that the principle of oneness is so encompassing that it goes beyond the barriers of time and space!

A WORD OF CAUTION: Whether you try it with live or dead people, cleansing, grounding and protection can never be over-emphasized. You would do better not to actively engage in such activity -- unless you are at peace with yourself, have proper cleansing and responsible guidance, and you are motivated by the highest desire to help others!

LIST HERE PEOPLE YOU WISH TO HELP HEAL:

CHAPTER 8

HAPPY ENDING

<u>The mystic powers of this book</u>

This is not a mere story book. It is not simply a book about healings. IT IS A HEALING BOOK! Already people involved with this book have experienced extra opening of THE EYE.

Keep it nearby at all times. Let your friends read it, but don't lend it out. Buy them other copies, but keep this one as a protective companion. Read it over and over again, and experience the results!

Joyful rebirth and rejuvenation with mature awareness

As you re-read this book, believe and know that you are rejuvenating yourself. With every new realization you achieve, know that you are reborn spiritually. While your body gets stronger and younger, your awareness is maturing. You are accumulating learning experiences which obviate painful "mistakes."

Letting the kids play happily and creatively

In this Aquarian Age, many of us are, indeed, in touch with the process of rejuvenation. The prerequisite to experiencing rejuvenation, or at least retarding aging, is to keep the natural child within our souls playing freely, happily and creatively. Some humor, some mischievousness, some blind trust, some unconditional Eros , some fantasy -- will go a long way to promoting Wholistic health and joyous longevity.

Writing your own book and script and sharing consciousness

Finally, I urge you to record your spiritual growth. As you express your thoughts and feelings the creative energies will flow through you like a fresh spring from the fountain of youth, cleansing and revitalizing your total being.

Keep notes, make tape recordings, write your own book! Use the scripts of your personal inspirations as aids in your own meditation.

Then share your expanded consciousness with others, as I have shared mine with you... Shalom.

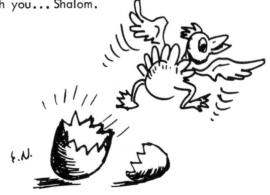

LAST-MINUTE GOOD NEWS FROM THE HOLY LAND!

As this revised edition goes to print, exciting news has arrived from Israel: My own mother, who is one of the cases discussed in the book, had another - and more dramatic - "miraculous" healing.

For years she had been resisting me - her son the healer - and "testing" my faith and perseverence, with her disbelief and disparagement. Time and again, with God's help, my students and I had "forced" a healing on her, and saved her physical body from dying. She had developed what was diagnosed as terminal cancer, in the form of tumors all over her body. Her physicians and most of her friends and family had given her up as lost, long time ago. Each time she was "forced" to heal, her conscious- ness again would resume the destruction of her cells, and she would take sick some time later.

So in December 1981, when I was urged by my mother and family to rush to Israel to say goodbye to her, if she lasted till I arrived, I decided: "No more fights with my mother! If she wants to die, I'll let her!" In- stead, I decided to work on her consciousness.

We discussed death and the after death. We explored the pros and cons of living and dying. We both worked on accepting my mother in the past, present, and future -- without judgment or expectation. And I helped her consider that when she was painfully throwing up and rapidly losing weight, she was ridding herself of her burden, toxin of all kinds, and negativity.

A day before my departure to the USA, I was compelled to disobey my mother's strict admonition not to talk with her physician so that I "don't confuse her with my nonsense." Well, Dr. Shakham, my mother's chief doctor, came to the phone immediately. The young lady physician listened attentively to my "nonsense" which had so embarrassed my mother. Frankly she admitted she was not familiar with any modalities of healing other than those she had learned in medical school. But confused she certainly was not. In fact, she promised to study my book WHOLISTIC HEALING with an open mind, and not to give up on my mother.

When instead of using her last ounce of strength to spank me in rage, my dear mother agreed to deliver WHOLISTIC HEALING to Dr. Shakham, I knew that something was moving inside her consciousness. I felt this was a good omen. And indeed my mother survived my visit, and was left thinking, feeling, suffering, and releasing...

On my way to Los Angeles, I was at peace. I knew that when my mother dies, she would make her transit more happily -- with less "garbage", and with much more awareness. I felt that this would be a healing, too: a healing of her soul. But I was also reminding myself of what I was telling my brothers, Oded and Doron, my father, and the doctors: "Don't bury her yet! She may not have yet fulfilled all of her good purpose in life. A miracle CAN happen - and why not to a healer's mother?!"

Sara, my devoted Jewish mama, kept shedding her layers of defensiveness, her attachment to things, and people, and life...her separations from God and good. She was letting go, letting go, letting go...I could see that in her letters, in my dreams, and in my meditative visits with her. With amazement and awe I was witnessing how, as my always tough and stubborn mother was weakening and mellowing and wasting away, I was feeling increasingly freer and more powerful and effective. And I was in touch with feelings of guilt about such a tragic blessing.

So I peered into the Torah and the Kabala, and deep into my consciousness, for answers to this mystery of life and death, losing and gaining, giving and receiving, surrendering to death and winning life. I began talking with God after midnight, and further experimented with long-distance communications and healing.

After much contemplation and months of meditation and prayer, I called my parents on their anniversary. I was the one who received a great gift! Mother's cheerful voice on the other side announced that she could not explain what was happening, but that she was feeling better than she had felt for the past few years. And yesterday, a couple of months later, my best "typical comments from readers" have arrived just in time to go to press. The words are not earthshakingly enthusiastic, but coming from my doubting, resisting mother, they a r e a m i r a c l e o f h e a l i n g and a beginning of something wonderful for many of us. Mother writes - and I'm translating from the Hebrew - "MY HEALTH HAS IMPROVED A GREAT DEAL, AND I BEGIN TO CREDIT IT TO THE MEDITATION AND PRAYER YOU CONDUCT MAY IT HELP." And my father, Jacob, writes, "Mother functions beautifully and everybody asks from where came the improvement!! Thank God, perhaps those prayers of yours, Elan!!!" (The exclamation marks are his!)

This letter, sealed, was delivered yesterday in person by special visitors from Israel, Ruth and Zvi, the parents of my sister in law Irit. They expressed their wonder about how mother, who was wasted down to less than 100 pounds, suddenly gained 17 pounds, rose from her deathbed, and regained her strength to such an extent that one would not even susspect she was ill.

As I am crying with joy, I have just resolved to write WHOLISTC HEALING II. The book will be dedicated to all my students in life, those who loved me and those who resisted me - especially to the latter, and especially to my mother - as they forced me to rely upon myself and God to find better paths.

Whether my mother Sara lives to read WHOLISTIC HEALING II, or departs earlier, she will live in the pages of the book as long as it is around helping and inspiring people.... because this is clearly part of her mission in life and in illness, and because in WHOLISTIC HEALING II I'll divulge some of my most personal healing and parapsychological techniques gifted to me to help mother, so that others can help themselves and their loved ones.

Praying that mother will stay around for a long time, I can envisage her transforming. I can envisage her dropping the "heaviness" she carried around, and thus allowing her beauty of person and soul to shine forth even more brightly. I can see her generosity and intelligence flowing unhindered, and her rich feelings freely experienced and expressed.   Whether in the flesh or in the hereafter, I can see her becoming an even more important instrument of light and love. I can see her initiated to the highest spiritual level that her Biblical name Sara - princess - implies and inspires. Amen!

ACKNOWLEDGEMENTS

Special thanks go to Su Su Levy - singles' ad writer and matchmaker- for her insightful assistance, and to Star Carter and Rena Burstein (now Elliott) for their devoted secretarial-plus help. Rena Elliott - my former student, trainee and assistant - deserves additional thanks for transforming in front of my eyes to become a successful psychic helper of people, and radio and TV personality--- thus demonstrating again that all this "stuff" really works; and for encouraging and helping me put this book on tape for the blind and for all who wish to HEAR WHOLISTIC HEALING .

My grattitude goes also to all my students, readers, and friends who suggested corrections and improvements of the book. Though too many to list in full, perhaps a special mention is due to my student Rita Rabin of UDC, for her scrutinizing proofreading; to Richard White - spiritual school headmaster - for his profound editorial suggestions on the revised edition; to Betty Paramore, for her wholistic and great assistance with the production of the revisions; and to Marilyn Yudelevitch, for her assistance with the "about the author" on the back cover, and for her intellectual, spiritual, and inspirational support of the revised edition.

REACHING HUMANITY IN MANY LANGUAGES
Numerous readers have requested to have *Wholistic Healing* available in other tongues, such as Hebrew, Arabic, Spanish, French, German, Russian, Japanese & Chinese. Translators & foreign publishers, you are warmly welcome to contact us with offers.

IN BRIEF
ABOUT SELF IMPROVEMENT INSTITUTE
Directed by Dr. Elan Z. Neev (Ph.D & DD)

RATIONALE: Sii teaching is not a dogma, religion or technique. It is, rather, a New Age process of natural growth from within you, according to your needs, capabilities, potentials, evolution, and roots. Focus is on your achieving a continuous flow with life's spontaneity--independent of teacher, technique, or theory.

GOALS: To foster harmony with life and fulfillment for the individual and society; for inner peace and world peace.

HIGHLIGHTS OF THE SELF-IMPROVEMENT ONENESS PROCESS:

* Powerful fusion of the best in New Age growth and awareness with Kabala secrets, channeled through Dr. Neev, in accord with the readiness of the individual and the group consciousness.

* Regression and progression for loving liberation from limitations on all levels to realize oneness and fulfill our missions.

* Energy linkage with the Highest, and synergy for God-given power to perform "miracles."

* Multi-sensory, multi-dimensional balancing through sound, color, breath, movement, and more --futuristic and ancient techniques.

* Practical integration and application of all knowledge, including nutrition, art, science, and metaphysics, for goal achievement, and to prevent or heal "spiritual indigestion."

* Safe acceleration of energies, to manifest peace, healing, abundance, love, joy, wisdom...and to be ready for the Great Changes.

* Taped review and conditioning.

MEMBERSHIP: Member of Association of Humanistic Psychology;
operating on a non-profit basis.

IF YOU WANT MORE...
STAY IN TOUCH!

HERE IS HOW:
You may call me to leave a message at 213/933-NEEV or
310/ **420-2072**, 9 to 9:30 in the morning is best. If long distanc
be prepared to be called back collect, or simply write to:
**Elan Z Neev, Director of ISI (previously SII),
P.O.Box 6300, Beverly Hills, CA 90212-1300**

* *
SUGGESTIONS TO FACILITATE A MORE SPEEDY REPLY

1) Type your letter, or at least write very legibly. State your purpose clearly right in the beginning.

2) Give your full name and address (if handwritten, please PRINT)
plus your day and evening phone numbers. It may help us to know
you better if you also include your birthdate, occupation, and--
in case you reside in a small town -- what city it is near. You ma
even include a small, recent photo of yourself with your name and
address printed on the back (You have mine; why shouldn't I have
yours?!).

3) Include a large (legal size at least) self-addressed envelope with
sufficient stamps for two ounces (My accountant will love you for
this!). *

WHY CONTACT ME?
1) To get a free listing of our self-improvement and healing tapes an
of our other Ageless Books publications (some exciting titles, as
you'll see!).

2) To get our latest schedule of events and an application for Sii classes (some of my sessions are free! !).

3) To purchase at cost (include $1) our comprehensive publication lavishly entitled ALMOST ALL YOU WANTED TO KNOW ABOUT SII, THE ONENESS PROCESS, AND DR. NEEV; AND WHAT THEY CAN DO FOR YOU -- AND WERE NOT AFRAID TO ASK! It will give you ample details about our classes, methods, rationale... and will feature some articles from local and national papers. It may provide you with some priceless ideas, and also will help you decide whether you want to study with me, or even work with me.

4) If you want private consultations in person, by phone, by mail, or in absentia through distant healing and prayer, tell me what you desire and you'll receive details about how to go about it.

5) If you want to host me as a speaker or presenter (I get along with most religious, social, professional, and political groups -- and with all ages and sexes).

6) If you wish to work as a volunteer or apprentice and receive by giving. Work can involve transcribing taped lectures and radio and TV shows, typing, editing, mailing, hosting events, distributing and posting flyers, telephoning, organizing, cleaning, and helping clients. Sii's future teachers, trainers and permanent staff will be chosen first from among graduates and volunteers.

7) If you desire to be involved in any way with our world peace projects, such as ICCWLWP (International Center of Communication for World Leaders and World Peace).

8) If you choose to work with us on an exchange basis or for sharing (commission basis), such as selling books and tapes and organizing seminars.

9) If you want us to help you raise funds for a worthy cause (such as your church, synagogue, or service organization) through an

entertaining, inspiring, and informative program, custom made to your specific requirements. I can MC and moderate, too.

10) If you need to tell me how much you hate or love me. In fact, I would love to hear your opinion about the book and what it is doing for you, for:

a) research purposes
b) improving what I give my readers and students
c) sharing your feelings and opinions with others so they will be inspired to help themselves and others.

PLEASE MAKE IT EASY to r e a d (see suggestions "1" and "2"). Unless you state otherwise, i t i s a s s u m e d t h a t y o u r c o m m e n t s m a y b e s h a r e d w i t h o t h e r s, orally and in print.

Eager to know you and by now your friend (hopefully),

teaching - you name it - we are certain you'll find this treatment invaluable. Some people may use it to retard aging and senility, and some to enhance their love life and sexual performance! **Side B: Confidence and Clear Mind** - A mind and soul decongestant, this treatment is great for your overall balance. It's a priceless tool for preparation for any task or challenge, mental, emotional, spiritual or physical. Athletes, performers, speakers, examination takers, and lovers should not be without it!

Tape 8: Side A: Losing Weight and Reshaping - There is a totally safe way to control your weight and shape. Dr Neev employs this safe way for results. But you do need to play this tape every night and morning for at least one month. **Side B: Overcoming Smoking** - This is a great way to overcome any bad habit, not just smoking. But for smokers it may be a lifesaver. And non-smokers, give it as a gift to someone who blows smoke in your air.

Tape 9: The Grand Journey - Available only for graduates of Dr Neev's Oneness Celebration Process (also the 40-hr and the 60-hr Intensives).

Tape 10: A: Parapsychological Beauty Treatment - You can see immediate results with this amazing natural beautifier! Look at yourself in the mirror before taking the treatment, or have your photo taken. Then look at yourself after taking the treatment, or take another photo and compare. Male or female, this fascinating beautifier/rejuvenator is also very, very good for your health...from the inside out! **Side B: World Peace Meditation** - It feels so good to contribute toward world peace and harmony, and every little bit of push in that direction helps. This is a recording of an actual world peace meditation conducted by Dr Neev in his pyramid Room. Meditating with this tape is a good way to join hands with Dr Neev's powerful group of planet healers. It can be an effective way to

be healed, too.

Tape 11: From Inner Peace to World Peace - World peace can help you maintain and improve your inner peace, and vice versa. If you feel the connection and would like to live with high New Age energies, you may appreciate this inspiring and interesting experience given by Dr Neev at *The New Age Awareness Fair* in San Francisco.

Tape 12: Heavenly Music Performed By Dr Neev - By popular demand, for healing, transformation and pleasure thru sympathetic resonance. **Side B: Love Projection for Wholistic Success and Good Luck** - Make love to life and it will follow you with "goodies " every where. Learn to "seduce" life and it will stay with you.

Tape 13: Side A: Compulsive Eating Overcome - Powerful friend to help you be in charge of you! **Side B: Changing Bad Habits - Truly!** Replace bad habits with desired habits that satisfy the same needs. The change is gentle; not thru brutal discipline.

STUDY & REVIEW *WHOLISTIC HEALING* ON TAPE:
By popular demand, you can now enjoy Dr Neev's book *Wholistic Healing* on tape for playing in bed, car, in gatherings and for the blind. Dr Neev's healing voice conducts the processes and meditations in the book as well as describes the illustrations. The rest of the book is read by the pleasant voice of the psychic healer Rena Elliott. An efficient way of studying and reviewing the life-giving and life-enriching techniques and inspiration of *Wholistic Healing* - even in your sleep.

TO ORDER *WHOLISTIC HEALING* BOOK ON TAPE:
If not available from your bookstore, you can get the entire set of 6 tapes for only $49 plus $3.50 for shipping and handling , plus the appropriate sales tax for your state. Buy it for

yourself or as a gift of life and love for someone who needs it.

TO ORDER *WHOLISTIC HEALING* 16-TAPE ALBUM AT A GREAT SAVINGS: *Wholistic Healing Book on Tape* PLUS *Wholistic Healing tapes* 1 thru 11, previously described, are conveniently & safely packed in a sturdy & attractive album that can be easily carried or stored like a book. It makes a wonderful & practical gift for yourself or dear ones...for life! Individually the tapes are valued at $10.90 each, total of $174.40, and the album at $10 - a grand total of $184.40. Add to it shipping, handling & tax, and the cost is well over $200. Until further notice, if you act now, you can get this life-saving, soul enriching album for only $180 including EVERYTHING!

JUST FOR YOU, INDIVIDUALLY - CUSTOM- MADE TAPES FOR YOUR SPECIAL NEEDS:

If you want the very best to suit your specific needs & your unique personality & soul, you can contract Dr Neev to create a tape just for you. Dr Neev will then prepare the tape individually & personally, based on his intuitive diagnosis of you & of what you request & need. To order, send a typed or VERY legibly written ONE page brief & clear description of your need or problem. Include your name, address, telephone & birth date.

If Dr Neev is to devote to you all the time needed to do a profound & effective job, it can take a lot of his time. The cost for the custom-made tape is $180 one side or $200 for a two-sided personal message & treatment, EVERYTHING included.

If you make good use of it playing it over over again to manifest what you need - healing, peace, love, objective achieved, etc. - it is like having Dr Neev's private session at your beck and call for life...very inexpensively. For each additional copy of the same tape, add $5.

For an additional **custom-made personal** tape addressing another objective or problem - separately - ordered at the same time, the cost is half ($90 for one side; $100 for both). For a custom- made tape **for another person** - ordered at the same time - deduct 10% from the 180 or 200 price.

SAFETY IS NO ACCIDENT - **A TAPE THAT CAN LITERALLY SAVE LIVES:** Are you concerned about drive-by shootings, car jackings, burglary, violence, riots, gangs, earthquakes, tornados, flood, fire, epidemics, airplane or car accidents, etc., etc., etc.? This tape can relieve much anxiety & practically reduce by far your statistical chance of getting hurt. Psychological, parapsychological, hypnotic & martial arts techniques work to improve your luck & protection. It's a magical and natural "insurance policy" that makes life easier. & it also turns you into a better driver & a safer passenger! $10.95 plus $2 shipping & handling plus the appropriate tax.

AGELESS BOOKS BY DR NEEV:

(1) Cosmic Doodlings for Self-Realization & Self-Coloring - A delightful book of drawings & cartoons to entertain, educate, inspire & guide. Through the eyes of Dr Neev's inner innocent & Godly child, your inner child is shown the best from all paths & religions, coupled with Dr Neev's original inspiration & creativity. (For the Christian fundamentalist, don't worry, by *Self*-Realization, Dr Neev means *God* Realization. Don't let semantics tempt you to sin by falsely judging. So it's "Kosher"!)

You can interact with it by coloring it, or by using it as a tool of "bibliocasting" (like bibliomancy) - choosing "at random" a page & analyzing what's the message for you or another. If a picture is worth a thousand words, these illustrations are worth countless thousands. It's a wonderful gift for any kid of any age & any background - two to 120! $6.95 plus $2 for shipping & handling plus the appropriate tax.

(2) The Art, Science & Magic of

Making Peace Happen: The Idealistic/Realistic Approach to Inner Peace & World Peace - This is a comprehensive manual of conflict resolution on all levels, and especially of how to live harmoniously even with differences. It's a thesis about how to apply the principles of unity in diversity. It's an original work about peace without pacifism...about peace & healing...about peace & martial arts...about Dr Neev's concept of *Organic Peace* that can really work! It includes some surprises & documentation about Dr Neev's connection with world leaders.

It informs, challenges...it even "pushes some buttons". It boldly discusses Hitler & Buddha, Carl Marx & Rabbi Nahaman & many other interesting & influential personalities. It's a process that will expand your tolerance level & global awareness...if you survive studying it from cover to cover. And it explains Dr Neev's vision of the International Center of Communications for World Leaders & World Peace. $14.95 plus $3 for shipping & handling, plus the appropriate tax.

AGELESS BOOKS BY DR NEEV TO BE AVAILABLE SOON (by the time you read this, they may be already available at book stores or from Dr Neev):

(a) *How to Break Thru Your Limitations* - A tiny book with a big, powerful message that can inspire & instruct you with proven techniques of smashing barriers & achieving success. $3.95 plus $1.50 for shipping & handling, plus the appropriate tax.

(b) *How to Feel Better* - It won't take you long to study this condensed, brief book, and it won't take long to see results either, if you apply what you've learned. It can affect profoundly the quality of your life in all areas, including how you feel emotionally & physically. It's both informational & inspirational. After completing the first draft in a heat of inspiration, Dr Neev "needed" to get severely ill so that he would have a chance to further investigate means of feeling better & include them in the book to help you in a very personal & compassionate way.

A wonderful gift for yourself, and get many extra copies to give dear ones. Price not determined yet at the time of writing this, but be assured it is very affordable & priceless!

(c) *God the Generous Capitalist: How to Borrow All You Need From the Cosmic Bank of Infinite Abundance* - This is a very essential book to perfect your consciousness in order to tap into endless riches. It is a must for anyone who wants to give more to life & to receive more from it. Like most of Dr Neev's Ageless Books, it is both profound and very, very practical...Price not determined yet at the time of writing.

AGELESS BOOKS & TAPES' SALES, GUARANTEE & RETURN POLICIES:

1) Dr Neev prefers that individuals buy his work from **bookstores and/or direct mail organizations** when available. Bookstores are urged to purchase his work from his **distributors**. If you are not able to get his work that way, you may order directly from Dr Neev. Allow three weeks for delivery. To expedite, send payment by money order & include a shipping label with your address.

2) In such a case you may deduct 10% of your total purchase price & shipping if you purchase more than 3 items (books, tapes, albums & sets); 20% on quantities of 10 or more items. None of the discounts are valid with other discounts. Each album or a set of tapes is counted as one item & already reflects a quantity discount in its price.

3) Books & tapes purchased by individuals from Dr Neev are **guaranteed** for one year. If after faithful use & application of his books & tapes for one year, you determine that you

wasted your money, send the items in question back to Dr Neev with the original **DATED** shipping envelope or package included, the cancelled check or a copy of it, and the accounting of how much you paid for each returned item. While you'll receive your purchase price for any reason, please state briefly & clearly your reason so that a lesson might be learned from it for the benefit of all. Your return for refund will only be honored if it's returned within 30 days after the one year guarantee since you received it...not earlier; not later. For merchandise bought from other suppliers, please deal with them & their policies, if return is needed.

ADDRESSES FOR ORDERING:
a) **Bookstores**, order from your distributors. Presently *New Leaf* of Atlanta, Georgia carries some of *Ageless Books & Tapes* publications.

b) **Individuals**, order from your bookstore or direct mail seller.

c) **Individuals & bookstores that cannot get** certain books, tapes & audiotapes of Dr Neev or *Ageless Books & Tapes* --- and any distributors, please order directly from:

> ELAN Z NEEV, DIRECTOR OF *AGELESS BOOKS & TAPES*, 4128 LAKEWOOD DRIVE, LAKEWOOD, CA 90712.

In case of unknown change in this direct & expedient address, please order from the permanent alternate address at P.O.BOX 6300, BEVERLY HILLS, CA 90212.

SPEEDING IT UP: At least two of your own address labels & your phone number, if included in your CLEAR order or inquiry, will facilitate speed of response. Self-addressed stamped envelope in addition to your phone number, will further insure quicker reply to your correspondence (we are busy, busy, busy!).

Wholistic Healing & Aromatherapy (A special Addendum):

"Wholistic healing embraces any modality that works, especially natural modalities of healing. Aromatherapy is one special natural ancient & rediscovered modality that has proven itself wonderfully. It requires much more space & attention than is within the scope of the book *Wholistic Healing*. I recommend that you explore it further by reading the following & availing yourself to more information & direct aromatic experience thru the use of essential oils." ..... Elan Z Neev

As ancient as the beginning of time, as modern as this moment, and as futuristic as eternity, AROMATHERAPY is truly a Divinely Provided modality for Wholistic Healing. The vital essences from the plant kingdom were given to us to balance and heal our bodies, minds and souls, ALL AT THE SAME TIME!! When we become imbalanced, "disease" (dis-ease) is manifest. This manifestation may be on a physical, emotional or spiritual level, but since all of these levels are interconnected, we must heal the situation by treating ALL levels. And, for this purpose, simultaneous balancing on all levels, we were provided with natural essential oils.

Each essential oil, derived from aromatic plants, flowers, roots, grasses, herbs and fruits, has specific properties which act on corresponding levels in the same manner. Just smelling the aromas releases a whole series of events that can result in **Complete** healing of our body, mind and soul. The scents go directly to the brain which signals the actual physical production of substances the body needs to heal itself. It is as if our internal pharmacy is triggered by the smell of certain aromas as though a prescription had been written. This results in the automatic production and release of the body's own, natural defense mechanisms. Lavender, for example, will relieve burns, will cause the release of endorphins (the body's pain relievers) into the blood stream to relieve stress and get rid of anger, and it will also alleviate the illusion of separation from the Creator and the "Why-me- Lord?" syndrome. Orange, actually builds collagen in the skin, gives strength and courage emotionally and rebuilds our link and connection with the One Source.

If you would like to explore this wonderful, unique and totally natural modality of wholistic healing and learn how you can use aromatherapy as an alternative to manmade synthetic preparations for treating the mind, body and soul, please contact:

Joyce Carol, President
Au Naturel
POB 956
Topanga CA 90290
(310) 455-7068   (800) 864-3999

We offer the highest quality, pure essential oils and related products, plus correspondence courses, seminars, and aromatherapist certification programs. We would love to hear from you, to answer your questions and to share your success stories. We would be happy to give any information to help you begin or further your use of wholistic healing with aromatherapy!!